SELF-ASSESSMENT IN
PATHOLOGY

To my mother.

# SELF-ASSESSMENT IN
# PATHOLOGY

JACK CRANE
MB, BCh, MRCPath, DMJ (Clin et Path)
Senior Registrar, State Pathologist's Department, Northern Ireland
Special Lecturer in Forensic Medicine and Honorary Tutor in Pathology,
The Queen's University of Belfast.

BLACKWELL ·
SCIENTIFIC PUBLICATIONS
OXFORD · LONDON · EDINBURGH
BOSTON · PALO ALTO · MELBOURNE

© 1984 by
Blackwell Scientific Publications
Editorial offices:
Osney Mead, Oxford, OX2 0EL
8 John Street, London, WC1N 2ES
23 Ainslie Place, Edinburgh, EH3 6AJ
52 Beacon Street, Boston
    Massachusetts 02108, USA
706 Cowper Street, Palo Alto
    California 94301, USA
107 Barry Street, Carlton
    Victoria 3053, Australia

All rights reserved. No part of this
publication may be reproduced, stored
in a retrieval system, or transmitted,
in any form or by any means,
electronic, mechanical, photocopying,
recording or otherwise
without the prior permission of
the copyright owner

First published 1984

Photoset by Enset (Photosetting),
Midsomer Norton, Bath, Avon
and printed and bound
in Great Britain by
Biddles Ltd,
Guildford, Surrey

DISTRIBUTORS

USA
    Blackwell Mosby Book Distributors
    11830 Westline Industrial Drive
    St Louis, Missouri 63141

Canada
    Blackwell Mosby Book Distributors
    120 Melford Drive, Scarborough
    Ontario, M1B 2X4

Australia
    Blackwell Scientific Book Distributors
    31 Advantage Road, Highett
    Victoria 3190

British Library
Cataloguing in Publication Data

Crane, Jack
    Self-assessment in pathology
    1. Pathology—Problems, exercises,
    etc.
    I. Title
    616'.0076      RB119
    ISBN 0-632-01397-4

# Contents

        Preface, vii

        Introduction, ix

1–24   General pathology, 1

25–36   Cardiovascular disease, 13

37–48   Respiratory disease, 19

49–60   Gastrointestinal disease, 25

61–72   Liver disease, 31

73–80   Pancreatic and gallbladder disease, 37

81–92   Renal disease, 41

93–104   Male and female genital tract disease, 47

105–116   Endocrine disease, 53

117–128   Bone and joint disease, 59

129–136   Breast and skin disease, 65

137–148   Nervous system disease, 69

149–160   Haematology, 75

161–200   Miscellaneous questions, 81

# Preface

This book is primarily intended for undergraduate medical students preparing for examinations in pathology. Its aim is to provide a method of self-assessment, as well as giving students the opportunity to practice MCQ technique. It should be used in conjunction with a standard undergraduate pathology text and should assist the student in highlighting those topics which require further study, as well as encouraging critical thought and a more fundamental understanding of disease processes.

The questions cover both general and systematic pathology (including haematology) and most are of the multiple true/false format. A small number of questions are of the five-choice association type. As well as providing answers to the questions, short explanatory comments have also been included which students might find helpful. The standard of the questions is based on the pathology teaching and examinations at The Queen's University of Belfast.

While mainly intended for undergraduates, it is hoped that candidates taking the Primary examinations for the FRCS and MRCPath may find the questions useful for revision purposes.

It is a pleasure to acknowledge the help I have received from many colleagues in the preparation of this book. I am particularly indebted to those members of staff of the Department of Pathology and to Professor J. M. Bridges of the Department of Haematology, The Queen's University of Belfast, for reading the questions and offering helpful advice and criticism. To Professor T.K. Marshall, State Pathologist for Northern Ireland, I owe a tremendous debt of gratitude for his constant support and encouragement. I am very grateful to my secretary, Miss Deirdre Prior, for translating my scribbles into the typed manuscript. I also wish to record my appreciation to Blackwell Scientific Publications Limited and in particular to Richard Zorab for their assistance and co-operation. Finally I would like to thank the medical students at Queen's on whom I have tried so many multiple choice questions and who have never failed to offer their comments and criticisms.

Belfast 1984

# Introduction

**Format of questions**
Two types of questions have been used, the multiple true/false variety and five-choice association.

Multiple true/false question—an initial statement is followed by five completions. Each completion must be correctly identified as either 'true or false'.

Five-choice association—five lettered headings are given, and seven numbered words or statements are listed below. One of the numbered words or statements is matched to the most appropriate heading.

The answers and explanations are given on the next page.

It is important to appreciate that in multiple choice questions examinations marks are deducted for wrong answers and it is therefore inadvisable to guess. If you do not know the answer, leave the question out.

# General Pathology

1 **The following may adversely affect wound healing:**
   A  Vitamin C deficiency
   B  Ultraviolet radiation
   C  Anabolic steroids
   D  Zinc
   E  Ischaemia

2 **Type I hypersensitivity reaction:**
   A  Is mediated by homocytotropic antibodies
   B  Is exemplified by the Mantoux test
   C  May result in the release of vasoactive amines
   D  Results in degranulation of T lymphocytes
   E  May cause acute anaphylaxis

3 **Fat embolism:**
   A  Only occurs as a result of fractures of bones
   B  May be diagnosed by the detection of fat globules in the urine
   C  Usually occurs about 10 days after injury
   D  When fatal is usually because of pulmonary insufficiency
   E  May be a cause of disseminated intravascular coagulation

4 **Down's syndrome (mongolism):**
   A  Occurs in about 1 in 100 live births
   B  Is more common with increasing maternal age
   C  Is usually due to trisomy 21
   D  May be associated with increased risk of development of leukaemia
   E  Is associated with raised alpha-fetoprotein levels in the amniotic fluid

## General Pathology: Answers

**1**  A  True.   Vitamin C is important for the synthesis of collagen
   B  False.  Ultraviolet light seems to enhance wound healing
   C  False.  Anabolic steroids enhance wound healing. Corticosteroids however may interfere with granulation tissue formation
   D  False.  Zinc is an important component of many enzyme systems and enhances wound healing
   E  True.   Wounds with a poor blood supply heal slowly

**2**  A  True.   These antibodies are bound to cells
   B  False.  The Mantoux test is an example of cell-mediated (delayed-type) hypersensitivity
   C  True.   Including histamine, serotonin and slow-reacting substance (SRS-A)
   D  False.  Degranulation of mast cells occur
   E  True.   Characterized by smooth muscle contraction and capillary dilation. The condition may be fatal

**3**  A  False.  Extensive soft-tissue injury involving subcutaneous fat may result in fat embolism
   B  True.   Fat globules may be detected in the urine and also in the sputum
   C  False.  The condition usually develops within 3 days of injury
   D  False.  Death is usually due to cerebral involvement
   E  True.   Due to activation of thromboplastic substances in the blood stream

**4**  A  False.  It occurs in about 1 in 600–700 live births
   B  True.   Due to increase in non-disjunctions during germ cell formation
   C  True.   There is an extra 21 chromosome giving a karyotype 47 XX or 47 XY
   D  True.   Mongols have a threefold risk of developing leukaemia
   E  False.  Alpha-fetoprotein levels are not raised unless there is an open neural tube defect such as in spina bifida

5 **Necrosis. Match the most appropriate feature listed below with the type of necrosis:**
   A  Fat necrosis
   B  Muscle necrosis
   C  Caseous necrosis
   D  Fibrinoid necrosis
   E  Colliquative necrosis

   1  Cerebral infarction
   2  Acute pancreatitis
   3  Accelerated hypertension
   4  Amyloid
   5  Zenker's degeneration
   6  Tuberculosis
   7  Sarcoid

6 **Pigmentation of the skin is a feature of the following:**
   A  Peutz–Jeghers syndrome
   B  Melanosis coli
   C  Chlorpromazine therapy
   D  Neurofibromatosis
   E  Phenylketonuria

7 **The following definitions are correct:**
   A  Hyperplasia is the increase in size of an organ due to increase in size of its constituent specialized cells
   B  Metaplasia is a change in one type of differentiated tissue to another type of similarly differentiated tissue
   C  A hamartoma is a tumour-like malformation in which the tissues are arranged haphazardly, usually with an excess of one component
   D  A granuloma is a localized collection of Langhan's giant cells
   E  Dystrophic calcification is the deposition of calcium salts in dead or degenerate tissue but where there is no upset in calcium metabolism

8 **Recognized effects of irradiation on the body include:**
   A  Atrophy of the seminiferous tubules
   B  Ulceration and haemorrhage of the bowel wall
   C  Osteosarcoma of bone
   D  Leukaemia
   E  Pulmonary fibrosis

## General Pathology: Answers

**5** A 2    Acute pancreatitis. Due to escape of enzymes, including lipase, into the peritoneal fat
    B 5    Zenker's degeneration. Associated with severe infections, particularly typhoid fever
    C 6    Tuberculosis. Caseous material consists of degenerative tissue within granulomata
    D 3    Accelerated hypertension. This is associated with necrosis of arterioles especially in the kidney
    E 1    Cerebral infarction. This is due to liquefaction of dead cells

**6** A True.    There may be circumoral pigmentation associated with hamartomatous polyps of the intestine
    B False.    This condition is associated with brown pigmentation of the mucosa of the large bowel
    C True.    Prolonged therapy may result in pigmentation of the skin and eye
    D True.    Large pigmented macules may be found—*café au lait* spots
    E False.    There is usually marked pallor in this condition due to inhibition of melanin formation

**7** A False.    This is the definition of hypertrophy. Hyperplasia implies increase in number of constituent cells
    B True.    Squamous metaplasia may, for example, occur in the bronchus as a result of chronic irritation
    C True.    A common example is a cartilaginous mass found in the lung
    D False.    A granuloma is a localized collection of epithelioid cells with or without giant cells
    E True.    Calcification may occur following chronic inflammation, infarction, etc.

**8** A True.    Due to destruction of the spermatogonia
    B True.    This may cause perforation or the late formation of fistulae, adhesions, etc.
    C True.    Either following local irradiation or due to the deposition of radioactive elements in the bone
    D True.    Spinal irradiation for ankylosing spondylitis has been associated with increased risk of leukaemia
    E True.    This may lead to progressive respiratory insufficiency

## 9 In tuberculosis:
A Hilar lymph node involvement is a feature of post-primary infection
B Rich's focus is an apical focus of infection in the lung
C The primary focus is always in the lung
D The cellular reaction is composed principally of polymorphs
E A negative tuberculin test will never occur with active disease

## 10 Chromosome abnormalities:
A In Klinefelter's syndrome the usual karyotype is 47 XXY
B In Turner's syndrome the usual karyotype is 45 YO
C The YY syndrome may be associated with aggressive behaviour
D Cystic fibrosis is associated with trisomy 21
E May be found in some cases of chronic leukaemia

## 11 Amyloid:
A In the kidney may be a cause of renal vein thrombosis
B Is a mucopolysaccharide
C May be stained with thioflavine T
D May be a cause of atrial fibrillation
E May be a cause of malabsorption

## 12 Granulomata are classically associated with:
A Chronic pulmonary beryllium disease
B Ulcerative colitis
C Crohn's disease
D Sarcoidosis
E Syphilitic aortitis

## General Pathology: Answers

**9**    A    False.    Post-primary infection is associated with an apical focus in the lung
     B    False.    Rich's focus is a subcortical focus in the brain
     C    False.    Occasionally the tonsils or gastrointestinal tract is involved
     D    False.    Epithelioid granulomata containing giant cells are the hallmark of tuberculosis
     E    False.    A negative test may occur with an overwhelming infection or when there is deficiency of the immune system

**10**    A    True.    Occasionally, there may be XXXY or XXXXY karyotypes
     B    False.    This condition affects females and the usual karyotype is 45 XO
     C    True.    These individuals are usually very tall and may have mild mental defect as well as demonstrating violent aggressive behaviour
     D    False.    There is no chromosomal abnormality in this inherited condition
     E    True.    The Philadelphia chromosome in chronic myeloid leukaemia

**11**    A    True.    Possibly due to dehydration and raised fibrinogen levels
     B    False.    It is a fibrillary protein
     C    True.    Amyloid shows green fluorescence when examined under ultraviolet light
     D    True.    Due to deposition in the left atrium of the heart in the elderly
     E    True.    Due to deposition in the wall of the small intestine

**12**    A    True.    Granulomata composed of histiocytes and giant cells are found in the lung
     B    False.    Granulomata are not found in this form of inflammatory bowel disease
     C    True.    Granulomata may be found in the bowel wall and in the regional lymph nodes
     D    True.    They may be found in the lungs, spleen, lymph nodes and other organs
     E    False.    This is characterized by inflammation around the vasa vasorum leading to fibrous replacement of the media.

## General Pathology: Questions

13 Match the *most appropriate* cell listed below for each of the conditions:
 A Cerebral infarction
 B Malakoplakia
 C Hashimoto's disease
 D Parkinson's disease
 E Hodgkin's disease

 1 Askanazy cells
 2 Touton giant cells
 3 Reed–Sternberg cells
 4 Anitschkow cells
 5 Lewy bodies
 6 Compound granular corpuscles
 7 Michaelis–Gutmann bodies

14 The following are considered to be carcinogenic in humans:
 A Aflatoxin
 B Thorotrast
 C Type I herpes hominis virus
 D Type II herpes hominis virus
 E Vinyl chloride monomer

15 Hormone production is a recognized feature of many tumours. Match the *most appropriate* hormone or chemical with each of the tumours listed below:
 A Squamous carcinoma of lung
 B Granulosa cell tumour
 C Carcinoid tumour
 D Hepatocellular carcinoma
 E Neuroblastoma

 1 Oestrogen
 2 Parathormone
 3 ACTH
 4 Alpha-fetoprotein
 5 Chorionic gonadotrophin
 6 5-hydroxytryptamine
 7 Dopamine

16 Examples of chemical carcinogenesis include:
 A Aniline dyes and bladder carcinoma
 B Radio-iodine and thyroid cancer
 C Arsenic and skin cancer
 D Cobalt and lung cancer
 E Fluoride and colonic carcinoma

# General Pathology: Answers

**13**  
A 6    Compound granular corpuscles. These are microglia which ingest necrotic lipid material  
B 7    Michaelis–Gutmann bodies. These are macrophages containing basophilic laminated inclusions  
C 1    Askanazy cells. These are large, eosinophilic, thyroid epithelial cells  
D 5    Lewy bodies. These are eosinophilic inclusions in residual neurones in the substantia nigra  
E 3    Reed–Sternberg cells. These multinucleated cells are thought to be pathognomonic of Hodgkin's disease  

**14**  
A True.    This toxic metabolite of fungi is thought to be related to liver cell carcinoma in man  
B True.    This was used as a radiological contrast medium in the past and has been associated with the development of various types of liver tumours  
C False.    This usually causes mucocutaneous lesions such as the 'cold sore'  
D True.    This may be causally related to cervical carcinoma  
E True.    This may be a cause of haemangiosarcoma of the liver  

**15**  
A 2    Parathormone. PTH production by these tumours may lead to hypercalcaemia  
B 1    Oestrogen. This may cause endometrial hyperplasia and endometrial carcinoma  
C 6    5-hydroxytryptamine. This may cause the 'carcinoid syndrome' characterized by flushing attacks, diarrhoea and bronchospasm  
D 4    Alpha-fetoprotein. About 90 per cent of these tumours synthesize AFP which can be detected in the blood  
E 7    Dopamine. These tumours may also secrete adrenaline and noradrenaline  

**16**  
A True.    Due to the presence of beta-naphthylamine in the urine  
B False.    This is an example of the carcinogenic effect of radiation  
C True.    Prolonged contact may cause a squamous carcinoma  
D False.    The increased risk of carcinoma in cobalt mine workers is related to radioactive ores  
E False.    There is no known association between fluoride and colonic cancer

## 17 The following may be associated with an underlying malignancy:
A Dermatomyositis
B Membranous glomerulonephritis
C Thrombophlebitis migrans
D Pyrexia
E Generalized exfoliative dermatitis

## 18 Match the *most appropriate* condition with each of the tests listed below:
A Kveim test
B Widal test
C Casoni test
D Frei test
E Schick test

1 Tuberculosis
2 Diphtheria
3 Sarcoidosis
4 Infectious mononucleosis
5 Lymphogranuloma venereum
6 Hydatid disease
7 Typhoid

## 19 Recognized features of systemic lupus erythematosus include:
A Necrotizing arteritis
B Positive Wassermann reaction
C 'Haematoxyphil bodies' in cells
D Positive antinuclear antibodies
E Wire-looping of glomerular capillaries

## 20 Features of delayed-type hypersensitivity reaction include:
A Inhibition by antihistamines
B Presence of sensitizing antibodies in the serum
C Predominant mononuclear cell infiltration
D Anaphylaxis
E Maximal reaction between 24 and 72 hours

## 21 Macrophages:
A Are similar to blood monocytes
B Are not found in the liver
C May cause lysis of fibrin in the inflammatory exudate
D May fuse to form giant cells
E Usually survive for less than 12 hours

## General Pathology: Answers

**17** A *True.* About 25 per cent of cases are associated with an underlying visceral malignancy
B *True.* In adults, about 25 per cent are associated with malignancy, usually lung carcinoma
C *True.* Characterized by transient inflammation and thrombosis of veins. Associated with lung, pancreatic and gastrointestinal carcinoma
D *True.* Due to production of pyrogens by some tumours
E *True.* This may be associated with an underlying lymphoma

**18** A 3 Sarcoidosis. This test involves the intradermal injection of splenic homogenate from a known case of sarcoid
B 7 Typhoid fever. This test demonstrates a rising titre of serum agglutinins
C 6 Hydatid disease. This is the intradermal injection of sterile hydatid cyst fluid.
D 5 Lymphogranuloma venereum. This involves the intradermal injection of material from an infected case
E 2 Diphtheria. This test involves the intradermal injection of diphtheria toxin

**19** A *True.* Particularly blood vessels in the kidney and spleen
B *True.* A false positive WR occurs in some cases
C *True.* These are similar to LE cells found in blood and bone marrow
D *True.* These are positive in nearly all cases
E *True.* This is associated with a membranous glomerulopathy

**20** A *False.* Glucocorticosteroids have a non-specific inhibiting effect
B *False.* The reaction is cell-mediated
C *True.* Macrophages, lymphocytes etc. and later, epithelioid cells
D *False.* This is a feature of type I hypersensitivity reactions
E *True.* The reaction is usually not visible before 12 hours and maximal at 24–72 hours

**21** A *True.* Monocytes are phagocytic cells found in the blood
B *False.* Kupffer cells in the liver are macrophages
C *True.* By the release of enzymes such as lysozyme
D *True.* Multinucleated giant cells are derived from macrophages
E *False.* These cells may survive for an indefinite period

## 22 The cells involved in the acute inflammatory process are:
A  Fibroblasts
B  Mast cells
C  Epithelioid cells
D  Lymphocytes
E  Polymorphonuclear leucocytes

## 23 Chemical mediators of acute inflammation include:
A  Histamine
B  Lymphokines
C  Bradykinin
D  Prostaglandins
E  Cleavage products of complement

## 24 Cardiovascular involvement in tertiary syphilis may cause:
A  Aortic incompetence
B  Myocardial ischaemia
C  Myocardial gummas
D  Abdominal aortic aneurysm
E  Libman–Sacks endocarditis

## General Pathology: Answers

**22**
- A False. These are associated with the healing process
- B True. These secrete vasoactive substances such as serotonin
- C False. These are seen in chronic granulomatous inflammation, e.g. tuberculosis
- D False. These are important in chronic inflammation and in cell-mediated immunity
- E True. These are probably the most important cells in the acute inflammatory response

**23**
- A True. This causes vasodilation and increases vascular permeability
- B False. These substances have a role in cell-mediated immunity
- C True. This substance increases vascular permeability
- D True. These substances are released from neutrophils and increase vascular permeability
- E True. Some of these are chemotactic and also cause release of vasoactive substances from cells

**24**
- A True. Due to dilation of the aortic valve ring
- B True. Due to narrowing of the coronary ostia
- C True. These are unusual however
- D False. Aneurysms usually develop in the aortic arch
- E False. This is a feature of SLE

# Cardiovascular Disease

25  Aortic incompetence may occur in:
 A  Infective endocarditis
 B  Rheumatoid arthritis
 C  Gout
 D  Ankylosing spondylitis
 E  Dermatomyositis

26  Aneurysms. Select the most appropriate feature listed below which matches the type of aneurysm:
 A  Berry
 B  Dissecting
 C  Mycotic
 D  Syphilitic
 E  Charcot–Bouchard

 1  Intracerebral haemorrhage
 2  Infective endocarditis
 3  Inflammation around vasa vasorum
 4  Calcification of media
 5  Vascular hamartoma
 6  Cystic medial necrosis
 7  Subarachnoid haemorrhage

27  **Infective endocarditis:**
 A  Is due to *Streptococcus faecalis* in the majority of cases
 B  May cause Osler's nodes in the fingers
 C  May cause nodular haemorrhagic spots on the palms and soles
 D  Never occurs on healthy valves
 E  May cause glomerulonephritis

28  **In rheumatic heart disease:**
 A  Pericardial involvement is rare in the acute stage
 B  The mitral valve alone is affected in about 40 per cent of cases
 C  Interstitial pneumonitis may occur
 D  There may be endocardial scarring in the left atrium
 E  The Aschoff nodule is pathognomonic of rheumatic fever

## Cardiovascular Disease: Answers

25 A  True.   Due to damage to the aortic valve
   B  True.   Aortitis may occur with weakening of the wall and consequent incompetence
   C  False.  This condition is characterized by the deposition of urate in joints. The aorta is not affected
   D  True.   Aortic involvement occurs in some cases
   E  False.  This condition mainly affects the skin and skeletal muscle

26 A  7   Subarachnoid haemorrhage. Due to an aneurysm on the circle of Willis
   B  6   Cystic medial necrosis. Medial degeneration leads to an intimal tear and dissection of the aortic wall
   C  2   Infective endocarditis. Infective emboli may lodge in the vessel wall causing destruction and weakness
   D  3   Inflammation around vasa vasorum. This causes loss of elastic tissue in the media and weakening of the wall
   E  1   Intracerebral haemorrhage. Caused by rupture of these microaneurysms in intracerebral vessels in hypertensive patients

27 A  False.  About 75 per cent of cases are still caused by *Streptococcus viridans*
   B  True.   These are painful red lesions, possibly embolic in origin
   C  True.   These are known as Janeway spots
   D  False.  Healthy valves may be affected, particularly in acute or ulcerative endocarditis
   E  True.   Usually a focal segmental glomerular lesion

28 A  False.  Typically, a fibrinous 'bread and butter' pericarditis occurs
   B  True.   Mitral valve alone 40 per cent; mitral and aortic valves 40 per cent
   C  True.   There may be an inflammatory infiltrate in alveolar walls and a fibrinous precipitate in the alveoli
   D  True.   McCallum's patch. This is usually situated above the posterior cusp of the mitral valve
   E  True.   This is a focus of fibrinoid material surrounded or infiltrated by Aschoff-type giant cells and other inflammatory cells

## Cardiovascular Disease: Questions

**29 In Mönckeberg's sclerosis:**
A There is intimal degeneration and calcification
B The arteries of the arms and legs are usually affected
C There are usually marked ischaemic effects
D Calcification is a result of lipid deposition
E There may be ossification of the deposits

**30 The following are recognized causes of acute fibrinous pericarditis:**
A Coxsackie B virus
B Uraemia
C Congestive cardiac failure
D Cardiac surgery
E Systemic lupus erythematosus

**31 In the development of atheromatous plaques:**
A Accumulation of lipid in the media usually occurs
B There is proliferation of smooth muscle cells
C Endothelial injury may be an important initial event
D There is accumulation of connective tissue matrix
E Calcification of the plaque rarely occurs

**32 In the diagnosis of acute myocardial infarction:**
A Creatine kinase (CK) shows a peak elevation after 24–48 hours
B Gamma glutamyltransferase ($\gamma$ GT) is characteristically raised
C Raised aspartate transaminase (AST) levels are specific for cardiac muscle infarction
D Lactate dehydrogenase (LD) may remain elevated for several days
E A second rise in enzyme levels after return to normal may indicate extension of the infarct

**33 Rupture of the myocardium following infarction:**
A Characteristically occurs 36–48 hours after infarction
B May cause cardiac tamponade
C May cause a VSD
D Rarely involves the anterior wall of the left ventricle
E Is frequently a complication of aneurysmal dilation of the left ventricle

## Cardiovascular Disease: Answers

**29**
- A  False.  There is calcification of the media of the arteries
- B  True.   Usually the muscular arteries of the limbs
- C  False.  The lesions do not normally encroach on the lumen
- D  False.  The cause of the condition, although unknown, is not thought to be related to lipid deposition
- E  True.   Occasionally the calcified deposits undergo ossification

**30**
- A  True.   This can cause both a pericarditis and a myocarditis
- B  True.   Possibly due to accumulation of nitrogenous products in the pericardial sac
- C  False.  Cardiac failure may cause an effusion but not pericarditis
- D  True.   Incision of the pericardium may be followed by pericarditis, possibly autoimmune in origin
- E  True.   Lupus erythematosus cells may occasionally be found in the pericardium

**31**
- A  False.  The lipid accumulates in the intima
- B  True.   These cells form a significant proportion of the cell population of the plaque
- C  True.   This may result in the adherence of platelets which may stimulate plaque formation
- D  True.   Including collagen, elastic fibre proteins and proteoglycans
- E  False.  Calcification frequently occurs in the advanced plaque

**32**
- A  True.   This enzyme is usually the first to become elevated after infarction
- B  False.  This enzyme is characteristically elevated in liver disease
- C  False.  AST is widely distributed in heart, liver, skeletal muscle and may be elevated following damage to any of these tissues
- D  True.   This is useful if the patient is not seen immediately after the onset of infarction
- E  True.   Extension of the infarct or the development of congestive cardiac failure

**33**
- A  False.  Rupture characteristically occurs between the fifth and seventh day when the infarct is maximally soft
- B  True.   Due to accumulation of blood in the pericardial sac
- C  True.   Due to rupture of the ventricular septum
- D  False.  The anterior wall is most frequently involved
- E  False.  The tough fibrous tissue of the aneurysm wall rarely ruptures

## Cardiovascular Disease: Questions

**34** The following abnormalities occur in Fallot's tetralogy:
- A Pulmonary stenosis
- B Atrial septal defect
- C Left ventricular hypertrophy
- D Right ventricular hypertrophy
- E Anterior aorta

**35 Aneurysms:**
- A Syphilitic aneurysms most commonly form in the aortic arch
- B Berry aneurysms are most frequently found on the vertebral artery
- C Atheromatous aneurysms may cause renal ischaemia
- D Dissecting aneurysms may be associated with defects in the media of vessels
- E Arteritis affecting the vasa vasorum of the aorta is the principal cause of syphilitic aneurysms

**36** For the conditions listed, select the most appropriate lesion from the list below:
- A Essential hypertension
- B Infective endocarditis
- C Systemic lupus erythematosus
- D Buerger's disease
- E Marfan's disease

1. Pericardial milk spots
2. Roth spots
3. Floppy mitral valve syndrome
4. Calcification of sinus of valsalva
5. Hyaline arteriolosclerosis
6. Libman–Sacks endocarditis
7. Inflammation of neurovascular bundle

## Cardiovascular Disease: Answers

**34** A *True.* Usually the subvalvular type
B *False.* There is a ventricular septal defect
C *False.* The left ventricular wall is of normal thickness
D *True.* This produces a 'boot-shaped heart' on X-ray
E *True.* The aorta overrides the VSD and receives blood from both ventricles

**35** A *True.* Aortic arch followed by thoracic and abdominal aorta and then the main arch vessels
B *False.* The most common sites are the bifurcation of the middle cerebral artery and the anterior cerebral (including anterior communicating) artery
C *True.* Due to involvement of the renal arteries and possible occlusion by thrombus
D *True.* The principal underlying cause for dissection is cystic medial necrosis where the muscle and elastic fibres are fragmented and replaced by mucoid substance
E *True.* Arteritis affecting the vasa vasorum is classically seen in syphilitic mesaortitis

**36** A 5 Hyaline arteriolosclerosis. Hyaline thickening of the arterioles, particularly in the kidney, is classically seen in essential hypertension
B 2 Roth spots. These are areas of retinal pallor, possibly embolic in origin
C 6 Libman–Sacks endocarditis. Small flat granular vegetations are found in this condition, particularly on the mitral valve
D 7 Inflammation of neurovascular bundle. The inflammation extends beyond the artery wall to involve the vein and adjacent nerve
E 3 Floppy mitral valve syndrome. This is due to myxoid degeneration of the mitral valve

# Respiratory Disease

37 **In sarcoidosis:**
   A   There may be hilar lymphadenopathy
   B   Diagnosis may be confirmed by a Heaf test
   C   Schaumann bodies may be found within granulomata
   D   There is an increased incidence of lung carcinoma
   E   Honeycomb lung may develop in long-standing cases

38 **The following may cause pulmonary fibrosis:**
   A   Hamman–Rich syndrome
   B   Farmers' lung
   C   Paraquat
   D   Asbestos exposure
   E   Lobar pneumonia

39 **Carcinoma of the lung:**
   A   May be associated with asbestos exposure
   B   Is of the oat-cell type in about 80 per cent of cases
   C   May involve the pericardium
   D   May cause Cushing's syndrome
   E   May be multifocal in origin

40 **Bronchiectasis:**
   A   May be associated with Kartagener's syndrome
   B   May be associated with massive lymphoid infiltration in the lung
   C   Is a cause of amyloid disease
   D   Is associated with marked dilation of the alveolar ducts
   E   May be associated with fibrocystic disease of the pancreas

## Respiratory Disease: Answers

**37**
- A  True.  Involvement of the hilar lymph nodes is a feature of the early stages
- B  False. The Kveim test, an intracutaneous injection of inactivated sarcoid material, is used to confirm the diagnosis
- C  True.  These are laminated, calcified structures found within giant cells
- D  True.  Possibly due to immunological deficiency
- E  True.  Due to progressive pulmonary fibrosis

**38**
- A  True.  This condition, of unknown aetiology, is associated with diffuse interstitial fibrosis
- B  True.  Caused by the inhalation of hay contaminated by fungi
- C  True.  When ingested this substance causes necrosis of alveolar epithelium and subsequent fibrosis
- D  True.  Long-standing exposure causes progressive interstitial fibrosis
- E  True.  Associated with failure of resolution and subsequent organization of the inflammatory exudate

**39**
- A  True.  Asbestos exposure predisposes to bronchial carcinoma and mesothelioma
- B  False. The majority (about 40 per cent) are squamous in type
- C  True.  Causing a pericarditis or a haemorrhagic pericardial effusion
- D  True.  Due to ectopic ACTH production
- E  True.  Particularly the bronchiolar type

**40**
- A  True.  This syndrome is associated with bronchiectasis, sinusitis and situs inversus
- B  True.  This is follicular bronchiectasis thought to be due to infection with adenoviruses
- C  True.  Long-standing inflammatory disease is a recognized cause of amyloidosis
- D  False. The disease is characterized by dilation of the bronchi and bronchioles
- E  True.  Due to obstruction of bronchi by thick mucoid secretions which become infected

## 41 For the conditions listed, select the most appropriate answer from the list below:
A Asthma
B Sarcoidosis
C Oat-cell carcinoma
D Shock lung
E Pulmonary fibrosis

1 Asteroid bodies
2 Hyaline membrane formation
3 Corpora amylacea
4 Busulphan therapy
5 ADH secretion
6 Ghon focus
7 Curschmann's spirals

## 42 Recognized causes of pulmonary hypertension include:
A Atrial septal defect
B Multiple pulmonary emboli
C Mitral stenosis
D Pulmonary fibrosis
E Chronic left ventricular failure

## 43 Simple coal workers' pneumoconiosis:
A Is characterized by panacinar emphysema
B Is due to the presence of silicates in coal
C Predisposes to bronchial carcinoma
D May precede the development of progressive massive fibrosis
E When present for more than five years almost invariably causes cor pulmonale

## 44 Bronchiectasis:
A May result in renal failure
B Is usually associated with bronchial obstruction
C May follow measles infection in children
D May be caused by alpha-1-antitrypsin deficiency
E May cause squamous metaplasia of the bronchial epithelium

# Respiratory Disease: Answers

**41**
| | | |
|---|---|---|
| A | 7 | Curschmann's spirals. These are whorls of shed bronchial epithelium found in the sputum of asthmatics |
| B | 1 | Asteroid bodies. These are star-shaped structures found in giant cells in sarcoid granulomata |
| C | 5 | ADH secretion. Inappropriate hormone secretion is well recognized in oat-cell carcinoma |
| D | 2 | Hyaline membrane formation. This consists of cellular debris and fibrin and is found following damage to the alveolar epithelium |
| E | 4 | Busulphan therapy. This drug, used to treat leukaemia, may cause intra-alveolar fibrosis |

**42**
| | | |
|---|---|---|
| A | True. | There is a left to right shunt with increased pulmonary blood flow |
| B | True. | Due to obstruction of the pulmonary arterial tree |
| C | True. | Due to back pressure from the left atrium |
| D | True. | Due to progressive obliteration of the pulmonary vascular tree |
| E | True. | This is a passive phenomenon due to back pressure via the left side of the heart |

**43**
| | | |
|---|---|---|
| A | False. | There is focal emphysema in which the respiratory bronchioles are affected |
| B | False. | The condition is due to the accumulation of carbon in the lung |
| C | False. | There is no direct evidence to link coal workers' pneumoconiosis with lung cancer |
| D | True. | Progressive massive fibrosis is characterized by nodular fibrosis and destruction of lung parenchyma |
| E | False. | Simple pneumoconiosis usually only causes slight functional disability and does not significantly shorten the normal life-span |

**44**
| | | |
|---|---|---|
| A | True. | Long-standing cases may develop amyloidosis which may progress to renal failure |
| B | True. | Obstruction is probably the most important underlying factor in the development of bronchiectasis |
| C | True. | Usually due to lung scarring following antecedent childhood infection |
| D | False. | This however is a recognized cause of emphysema |
| E | True. | Due to long-standing bronchial irritation |

## 45 Influenza virus:
A Causes necrosis of the bronchial mucosa
B Predisposes to secondary bacterial infection
C Causes a reduction in bronchial secretion
D Is a myxovirus with a short incubation period
E Causes an acute bronchiolitis

## 46 Oat-cell carcinoma of lung:
A Is characteristically not radiosensitive
B Thought to be derived from cells of the APUD series
C Histologically shows the formation of keratin pearls
D Is related to some bronchial adenomas
E Arises from areas of squamous metaplasia of the bronchial epithelium

## 47 Pleural effusion may be associated with:
A Asthma
B Meigs' syndrome
C Mesothelioma
D Systemic lupus erythematosus
E Tuberculosis

## 48 Lobar pneumonia:
A Resolves by crisis after 3–4 days
B Grey hepatization is characterized histologically by alveoli filled with fibrin
C Is usually due to *Haemophilus influenzae*
D May be associated with alcoholism
E Is usually the result of blood-borne infection

## Respiratory Disease: Answers

**45** A *True.* The virus attacks columnar ciliated respiratory epithelium
B *True.* This is a serious complication of influenza infection
C *False.* There is increased bronchial secretion
D *True.* Its incubation period is about two days
E *True.* A peribronchial inflammatory reaction is typically seen

**46** A *False.* These tumours, although highly malignant, are highly radiosensitive
B *True.* These cells have the ability of amine precursor uptake and decarboxylation
C *False.* Keratin pearl formation is seen in squamous carcinomas
D *True.* Many bronchial adenomas are of the carcinoid type and are derived from APUD cells
E *False.* This probably applies to squamous carcinomas

**47** A *False.* This condition is one of bronchial narrowing. The pleura is not involved
B *True.* In this condition, ovarian fibromas are associated with a pleural effusion and ascites
C *True.* This malignant pleural tumour may cause a blood-stained effusion
D *True.* In SLE there may be pleural, pericardial and peritoneal involvement
E *True.* This is still one of the most common causes of a pleural effusion

**48** A *False.* Resolution classically occurs between the fifth and seventh day
B *False.* Fibrin is usually absent and the alveoli are filled with neutrophils
C *False.* 60–80 per cent of cases are due to *Streptococcus pneumoniae* (pneumococcus)
D *True.* Alcoholism, by causing generalized debility, is a recognized predisposing condition
E *False.* Infection occurs via the bronchial tree by inhalation

# Gastrointestinal Disease

**49 Ulcerative colitis:**
A  Is characterized by the presence of skip lesions in the bowel
B  Histologically may show the formation of crypt abscesses
C  Is associated with an increased risk of the development of intestinal lymphoma
D  Involves the rectum in less than half of all cases
E  May be associated with a raised serum alkaline phosphatase

**50 Crohn's disease:**
A  May be associated with non-caseating granulomata in the regional lymph nodes
B  May cause a positive Kveim test
C  Does not predispose to carcinoma
D  May cause malabsorption
E  Rarely causes fissure ulcers in the bowel

**51 Peptic ulcer:**
A  May occur in the terminal ileum
B  Occurs more commonly in the stomach than the duodenum
C  Does not occur with complete achlorhydria
D  Usually has a heaped-up craggy margin
E  May be secondary to severe head injury

**52 In coeliac disease:**
A  An increased incidence of gastrointestinal malignancy has been reported
B  The terminal ileum is principally involved
C  Biopsy of the intestine usually shows villous atrophy
D  There may be an association with dermatitis herpetiformis
E  There is an association with the HL–A8 antigen

## Gastrointestinal Disease: Answers

**49**  A  *False.*  The disease is not segmental but affects the bowel in continuity
    B  *True.*  These are crypts of Liberkuhn containing polymorphs, mucus, etc.
    C  *True.*  An increased incidence of lymphomas has been reported although the risk of developing a carcinoma is more important
    D  *False.*  The rectum is involved in virtually all cases
    E  *True.*  Due to associated liver involvement

**50**  A  *True.*  Granulomata may be found in the bowel wall and in draining lymph nodes
    B  *True.*  The Kveim is positive in about 50 per cent of cases
    C  *False.*  There is evidence that Crohn's disease predisposes to carcinoma of the small intestine
    D  *True.*  Due to involvement of the small intestine
    E  *False.*  Deep fissure ulcers are characteristic of Crohn's disease

**51**  A  *True.*  Due to ectopic gastric mucosa in a Meckel's diverticulum secreting acid
    B  *False.*  Duodenal ulcers are about three times more common than gastric ulcers
    C  *True.*  The presence of gastric juice appears essential for peptic ulcer formation
    D  *False.*  Such an appearance would be suggestive of malignancy
    E  *True.*  This is a Cushing's ulcer and is associated with increased acid output in the stomach

**52**  A  *True.*  Particularly the development of lymphoma and carcinoma of the small bowel and oesophagus
    B  *False.*  The upper jejunum is most severely affected
    C  *True.*  This is an important histological feature of the condition
    D  *True.*  About 60 per cent of patients with dermatitis herpetiformis have evidence of coeliac disease
    E  *True.*  HL–A8 antigen is found in about 80 per cent of patients

## 53 Recognized features in typhoid fever include:
A Cholecystitis
B Leucocytosis
C Ulceration of the small bowel
D Muscle necrosis
E Phagocytosis of red cells in the bowel wall

## 54 Chronic gastric ulcer:
A Greater than 4 cm diameter is invariably malignant
B Undergoes malignant change in about 10 per cent of cases
C Occurs most commonly on the lesser curve of the stomach
D Is usually associated with increased gastric acid secretion
E May cause pyloric stenosis

## 55 Gastric carcinoma:
A Is more common in patients with pernicious anaemia
B Occurs most commonly in the fundal area
C If confined to the mucosa and submucosa is termed 'early gastric cancer', regardless of lymph node metastasis
D May be associated with a desmoplastic reaction
E When it arises from a peptic ulcer usually develops from the crater base

## 56 Concerning the appendix:
A Rupture of a mucocele may result in myxoma peritonei
B May be a site of endometriosis
C Warthin–Finkeldey cells may be found in measles
D Is never involved in Crohn's disease
E Acute appendicitis may result in portal pyaemia

## 57 Carcinoma of the oesophagus:
A Is more common in females than males
B Is rare in individuals under 50 years of age in the United Kingdom
C Is common in heavy drinkers
D Occurs in the post-cricoid region in about 60 per cent of cases
E Is usually an adenocarcinoma

## Gastrointestinal Disease: Answers

**53** 
- A  True.   Residual cholecystitis may result in a carrier state
- B  False.  Characteristically there is leucopenia
- C  True.   Particularly in the terminal ileum
- D  True.   Toxic coagulation of skeletal muscle may occur (Zenker's degeneration)
- E  True.   Mononuclear cells in the gut phagocytose red cells and organisms

**54**
- A  False.  The size of an ulcer is a poor indication of malignancy
- B  False.  Probably no more than 1 per cent of gastric ulcers undergo malignant change
- C  True.   Ulcers are rarely found on the greater curve
- D  False.  Gastric acid secretion is usually normal but is increased in duodenal ulcers
- E  True.   Healing of an ulcer near the pylorus may cause pyloric narrowing

**55**
- A  True.   Three to four times more common in these patients. Related to intestinal metaplasia and atrophic gastritis
- B  False.  The majority arise in the pyloric region and antrum
- C  True.   This is the definition of early gastric cancer
- D  True.   This is the formation of a marked fibrous stroma in the tumour
- E  False.  Carcinoma arises from the epithelium at the ulcer margin

**56**
- A  True.   The peritoneal cavity becomes filled with gelatinous material
- B  True.   Foci of endometriosis may be found in the wall, particularly on the serosa
- C  True.   These giant cells are found in the lymphoid tissue
- D  False.  The appendix may be involved by itself or together with the ileum
- E  True.   As a result of septic thrombophlebitis and formation of septic emboli

**57**
- A  False.  It is approximately four times more frequent in males than females
- B  True.   The average age is about 65 years
- C  True.   It is about 25 times more common in this group
- D  False.  Only about 20 per cent occur in the upper oesophagus
- E  False.  About 90 per cent are squamous in type

**58 In Hirschsprung's disease:**
A Ganglion cells are only rarely absent from the distal rectum
B There is an increased incidence in females over males
C There is a frequent association with pyloric stenosis
D Presentation is usually with diarrhoea, vomiting and abdominal distension
E There is an increased incidence of pseudomembranous colitis

**59 The following are recognized causes of intestinal malabsorption:**
A Vitamin $B_{12}$ deficiency
B Whipple's disease
C Diverticular disease of the colon
D Tropical sprue
E Giardiasis

**60 The following predispose to carcinoma of the colon:**
A Villous adenoma
B Metaplastic polyp
C Melanosis coli
D Familial polyposis
E Ulcerative colitis

## Gastrointestinal Disease: Answers

**58** A *False.* Ganglion cells are always absent. The condition is thought to be due to failure of migration of the cells from the neural crest
B *False.* It is about 6–9 times more common in boys than girls
C *False.* Although it may be associated with other congenital abnormalities
D *False.* Presentation is usually with severe constipation
E *True.* The precise reason for this is not known

**59** A *False.* However malabsorption may affect the intestinal bacterial flora and *cause* vitamin $B_{12}$ deficiency
B *True.* This is a rare cause of steatorrhoea in middle-aged males in which bacilliform particles have been found in the lamina propria
C *False.* Since this does not affect the small intestine
D *True.* This is endemic in S.E. Asia. It is characterized by partial villous atrophy and inflammation of the lamina propria
E *True.* This may cause partial villous atrophy of the mucosa

**60** A *True.* This type of adenoma has a high malignant potential
B *False.* These polyps are not neoplastic and hence will not undergo malignant change
C *False.* This condition has no malignant potential. It may be caused by the ingestion of laxatives
D *True.* This condition, inherited in an autosomal dominant fashion, has a very definite malignant potential
E *True.* Definite risk of malignancy especially in patients with chronic continuous disease

# Liver Disease

61 **Fatty change of the liver:**
   A  May occur in diabetes
   B  May result from tetracycline therapy
   C  Occurs in Reye's syndrome
   D  May occur as a complication of pregnancy
   E  May follow intestinal bypass operations for obesity

62 **The following have an aetiological association with cirrhosis:**
   A  Alpha-1-antitrypsin deficiency
   B  Crohn's disease
   C  Alcohol
   D  Intestinal bypass surgery for obesity
   E  Budd–Chiari syndrome

63 **A 50-year-old alcoholic is admitted to hospital with jaundice. A liver biopsy shows the features of a micronodular cirrhosis. Which of the following might you expect to find:**
   A  Testicular atrophy
   B  Hypoalbuminaemia
   C  Raised gamma globulin level
   D  Splenomegaly
   E  Anaemia

64 **Primary (idiopathic) haemochromatosis:**
   A  Has an autosomal dominant mode of inheritance
   B  May result in testicular atrophy
   C  May predispose to hepatocellular carcinoma
   D  May be a cause of cardiac failure
   E  Accumulated iron in the liver may be stained with Congo red

65 **Acute hepatitis:**
   A  Type B may be transmitted sexually
   B  Type A has an average incubation period of 100 days
   C  Type A usually progresses to chronic hepatitis
   D  May be associated with Councilman bodies in the liver
   E  Type A may predispose to hepatocellular carcinoma

## Liver Disease: Answers

**61** A *True.* Particularly in older diabetics. It is not thought to have clinical significance
B *True.* Tetracyclines produce microvesicular fatty change
C *True.* This condition occurs in children and is characterized by encephalopathy and microvesicular fatty infiltration
D *True.* Acute fatty liver of pregnancy which progresses rapidly to hepatocellular failure
E *True.* This may be followed by hepatocellular degeneration, neutrophil leucocyte infiltration, fibrosis and cholestasis

**62** A *True.* This condition is also associated with emphysema
B *True.* Cirrhosis is 12 times more common in patients with chronic inflammatory bowel disease
C *True.* This is one of the most common causes of cirrhosis in the western world
D *True.* Probably due to hepatotoxins passing into the portal circulation
E *True.* In this syndrome there is hepatic venous obstruction

**63** A *True.* Due to failure to inactivate oestrogen
B *True.* From failure to synthesize plasma proteins
C *True.* Although the precise cause of this is not understood
D *True.* Due to portal hypertension
E *True.* Usually iron-deficiency type related to gastrointestinal haemorrhage and hypersplenism

**64** A *False.* It has an autosomal recessive mode of inheritance
B *True.* Due to the deposition of iron in the testes and to failure to inactivate oestrogen
C *True.* Usually after the development of cirrhosis
D *True.* Due to deposition of iron in the myocardium
E *False.* The Prussian blue stain is used. Congo red is used to stain amyloid

**65** A *True.* There is a high incidence in male homosexuals
B *False.* The incubation period is shorter, between 15 and 40 days
C *False.* Most cases of type A resolve completely
D *True.* These are degenerate liver cells which appear deeply eosinophilic
E *False.* There is no evidence to suggest this

# Liver Disease: Questions

**66 Causes of portal hypertension include:**
A  Schistosomiasis
B  Budd–Chiari syndrome
C  Constrictive pericarditis
D  Oesophageal varices
E  Ingestion of senecio alkaloids

**67 Primary biliary cirrhosis:**
A  Is more common in males than females
B  Usually occurs in the second and third decades
C  Is associated with elevated serum IgM levels
D  May be associated with Sjögren's syndrome
E  Histologically may show granulomata in the portal tracts

**68 In obstructive jaundice:**
A  Urobilinogen is increased in the urine if obstruction is complete
B  Serum alkaline phosphatase is increased
C  Serum gamma-glutamyltransferase is elevated
D  The stools are dark
E  The level of unconjugated bilirubin in the blood is markedly increased

**69 The following may be associated with the development of liver tumours:**
A  Oral contraceptive pill
B  Vinyl chloride monomer
C  Hepatitis B virus
D  Mycotoxins
E  Arsenic

**70 Widespread liver cell necrosis may be a complication of:**
A  Halothane exposure
B  Paracetamol overdose
C  Haemosiderosis
D  Polycystic disease of the liver
E  Hepatitis B infection

## Liver Disease: Answers

**66**
- A *True.* Due to periportal fibrosis
- B *True.* This is thrombosis of the hepatic veins
- C *True.* As a result of chronic venous congestion of the liver
- D *False.* This is a consequence, and not a cause, of portal hypertension
- E *True.* These alkaloids cause veno-occlusive liver disease characterized by occlusion of hepatic venous radicles

**67**
- A *False.* About 90 per cent of cases occur in females
- B *False.* Most patients are over 50 years of age
- C *True.* The disease has a probable immunological aetiology
- D *True.* This and other immune disorders may be found
- E *True.* These are usually found in the early florid stage of the disease

**68**
- A *False.* Urobilinogen is absent from the urine
- B *True.* This is indicative of cholestasis
- C *True.* This is elevated in many forms of liver disease particularly if there is cholestasis
- D *False.* The stools are pale since no bilirubin is excreted into the bowel
- E *False.* The level of conjugated bilirubin is increased

**69**
- A *True.* Women on long-term oral contraceptives have an increased risk of developing liver cell adenomas
- B *True.* Workers exposed to vinyl chloride monomer have an increased incidence of haemangiosarcoma of the liver
- C *True.* There is a significant association between hepatitis B virus infection and liver cell carcinoma
- D *True.* Aflatoxins, in particular, are thought to be associated with liver cell carcinoma
- E *True.* Arsenic may predispose to the development of haemangiosarcoma

**70**
- A *True.* Particularly following repeated exposure
- B *True.* This may cause centri-zonal necrosis
- C *False.* In this condition iron is deposited in the Kupffer cells
- D *False.* This condition does not cause liver necrosis. It may be associated with polycystic disease of the kidneys
- E *True.* This may cause massive necrosis and liver failure

# 71 Chronic active hepatitis:
A  May follow hepatitis A infection
B  May be a feature of Wilson's disease
C  May be associated with high serum antibody levels
D  Does not progress to the development of cirrhosis
E  Does not cause liver cell necrosis

# 72 Heavy alcohol consumption may cause:
A  Hepatic steatosis
B  Mallory's hyaline formation in the liver
C  Cardiomyopathy
D  Widespread granuloma formation in the liver
E  Iron deposition in the liver

## Liver Disease: Answers

**71** A *False.* However, hepatitis B and non-A non-B hepatitis are recognized causes
B *True.* This condition is due to the deposition of copper in the liver
C *True.* This is a feature of the 'lupoid hepatitis' form of chronic active hepatitis
D *False.* Cirrhosis develops in a substantial number of cases
E *False.* Piecemeal liver cell necrosis is an essential feature of the condition and may be extensive

**72** A *True.* This is fatty change of the hepatocytes
B *True.* This eosinophilic hyaline material is deposited in hepatocytes
C *True.* This may result in heart failure
D *False.* Granulomata are not a significant feature of alcoholic liver disease
E *True.* Probably due to drinking large quantities of wine

# Pancreatic and Gallbladder Disease

73 **Cystic fibrosis:**
   A  Is inherited as an autosomal dominant condition
   B  May be diagnosed by measuring the salt concentration of sweat
   C  May present as meconium ileus
   D  Is a recognized cause of biliary cirrhosis
   E  Is associated with repeated respiratory infections

74 **Carcinoma of the pancreas:**
   A  Shows a definite increased incidence in heavy drinkers
   B  Shows a definite increased incidence in heavy smokers
   C  Is usually an adenocarcinoma
   D  Usually occurs in the tail of the pancreas
   E  May be associated with raised levels of carcinoembryonic antigen

75 **Acute pancreatitis:**
   A  May be associated with hyperparathyroidism
   B  May cause a transient rise in blood calcium
   C  Usually only causes a slight rise in serum amylase
   D  May be caused by reflux of duodenal contents into the pancreatic duct
   E  Occasionally occurs in polyarteritis nodosa

76 **Gallstones:**
   A  May be caused by a mucocele of the gallbladder
   B  Have an increased incidence in patients with congenital spherocytosis
   C  Are usually composed of calcium carbonate
   D  Are formed in bile which is supersaturated with bile acids
   E  Are found in about 40 per cent of the adult population

## Pancreatic and Gallbladder Disease: Answers

**73** A *False.* The disease is transmitted by a single autosomal recessive gene
B *True.* Increased concentrations of sodium and chloride are found in the sweat
C *True.* Viscid mucus and meconium may cause intestinal obstruction in the neonate
D *True.* Due to obstruction of bile ducts by viscid bile
E *True.* Due to bronchial obstruction by viscid mucus

**74** A *False.* No definite association has been found
B *True.* It is 2–3 times more common in heavy smokers
C *True.* An adenocarcinoma usually with a marked scirrhous stroma
D *False.* About 60 per cent are found in the head of the pancreas
E *True.* About 90 per cent of patients are found to have raised serum levels of CEA

**75** A *True.* Increased levels of calcium in pancreatic juice may activate trypsinogen
B *False.* Serum calcium usually falls possibly due to deposition in areas of fat necrosis
C *False.* Typically the serum amylase is greatly raised (over 1000 i.u.)
D *True.* The pancreatic enzymes may be activated by duodenal secretions
E *True.* Due to ischaemic infarction of the pancreas

**76** A *False.* Mucocele is the result of obstruction of the cystic duct by stones
B *True.* Pigment stones form due to increased haemolysis of red cells
C *False.* About 90 per cent of stones are mixed (composed of cholesterol, bile pigment, calcium and protein)
D *False.* They occur in bile supersaturated with cholesterol
E *False.* They are found in about 10 per cent of the adult population

## 77 Carcinoma of the gallbladder:
A   Is characterized histologically by the formation of Aschoff–Rokitansky sinuses
B   Is usually an adenocarcinoma
C   Is usually associated with the presence of gallstones
D   Is more common in men than women
E   May be related to carcinogens in bile

## 78 Islet cell tumours of the pancreas:
A   May secrete gastrin
B   May secrete insulin
C   May be associated with parathyroid adenomas
D   Are usually benign
E   May cause hyperkalaemia

## 79 In pancreatic islet tissue:
A   Beta cells secrete insulin
B   D cells secrete calcitonin
C   Alpha cells secrete glucagon
D   Islet cells belong to the APUD series
E   Occasional Paneth cells are found

## 80 Primary sclerosing cholangitis:
A   Is usually caused by gallstones
B   May be associated with ulcerative colitis
C   May progress to biliary cirrhosis
D   Frequently results in the formation of a mucocele of the gallbladder
E   May be associated with retroperitoneal fibrosis

Pancreatic and Galbladder Disease: Answers

**77**
- A  False.  These are downgrowths of epithelium associated with chronic cholecystitis
- B  True.  About 90 per cent are adenocarcinomas although squamous carcinomas occur in a few cases
- C  True.  Gallstones are present in about 80 per cent of cases and are thought to be an important causative factor
- D  False.  It is about four times more common in females
- E  True.  Some derivatives of cholic acid, a bile component, are known to be potent carcinogens

**78**
- A  True.  Causing multiple recurrent peptic ulcers (Zollinger–Ellison syndrome)
- B  True.  Causing attacks of hypoglycaemia
- C  True.  Islet cell tumours may occur as part of the multiple endocrine adenoma syndrome
- D  True.  Over 80 per cent of these tumours behave in a benign fashion
- E  False.  Hypokalaemia however may occur due to severe diarrhoea from secretion of vasoactive intestinal peptide (VIP)

**79**
- A  True.  Beta cells form the bulk of islet tissue (60–70 per cent)
- B  False.  D cells secrete gastrin
- C  True.  Glucagon raises the blood sugar and secretion is stimulated by hypoglycaemia
- D  True.  The cells are derived from neuroectoderm and secrete polypeptide hormones
- E  False.  These are found mainly in the small intestine and occasionally in the stomach and large bowel

**80**
- A  False.  Acute obstructive cholangitis is usually due to bile duct obstruction by stones
- B  True.  There is a recognized association between these conditions
- C  True.  Associated with obliteration of bile ductules
- D  False.  A mucocele results from unrelieved obstruction of the cystic duct
- E  True.  Due to extension of the fibrotic process into the biliary tract

# Renal Disease

81 **Acute pyelonephritis:**
   A  Is more common in females than males
   B  Most first attacks are due to *Streptococcus faecalis*
   C  A bacteriuria of 10 000 organisms per millilitre of urine is significant
   D  Is usually due to blood-borne infection
   E  May cause ureteric obstruction

82 **Features of chronic renal failure may include:**
   A  Normochromic normocytic anaemia
   B  Respiratory acidosis
   C  Parathyroid hyperplasia
   D  Colitis
   E  Radiological opacities in the lungs

83 **Membranous glomerulonephritis:**
   A  Commonly presents as the nephrotic syndrome
   B  May be associated with an underlying malignancy
   C  Causes widespread epithelial crescent formation in the glomeruli
   D  May be associated with granular IgG and $C_3$ deposits in the glomeruli
   E  Usually carries an excellent prognosis

84 **Renal changes in diabetes include:**
   A  Armanni–Ebstein lesion
   B  Papillary necrosis
   C  Kimmelstiel–Wilson lesion
   D  Hyaline arteriolosclerosis
   E  Pyelonephritis

# Renal Disease: Answers

**81**
- A  *True.*  About 10 times more common in females
- B  *False.*  *Escherichia coli* is responsible for most first attacks
- C  *False.*  This might be due to contamination. A significant bacteriuria is >100 000 organisms per millilitre
- D  *False.*  Ascending infection from the bladder accounts for the majority of cases
- E  *True.*  Due to blockage with inflammatory material and necrotic debris

**82**
- A  *True.*  Possibly due to inhibited marrow action by toxic products or to decreased erythropoietin production
- B  *False.*  There is usually a metabolic acidosis due to impairment of bicarbonate generation
- C  *True.*  Retention of phosphate leads to urinary loss of calcium resulting in secondary parathyroid hyperplasia
- D  *True.*  Urea diffuses into the gut where it is acted upon by organisms to produce ammonia which causes mucosal irritation
- E  *True.*  Usually when the uraemic patient is hypertensive and in left ventricular failure

**83**
- A  *True.*  The majority of cases present with non-selective proteinuria
- B  *True.*  Particularly carcinoma of the lung and colon
- C  *False.*  Histologically, the disease is characterized by diffuse thickening of the basement membrane
- D  *True.*  Immune complexes are deposited towards the epithelial side of the GBM and within it
- E  *False.*  About 25 per cent of cases progress to renal failure

**84**
- A  *True.*  This is the deposition of glycogen in the tubular epithelium
- B  *True.*  Probably due to ischaemia from microangiopathy of renal vessels
- C  *True.*  This is nodular glomerulosclerosis and is characteristically seen in the diabetic kidney
- D  *True.*  This affects both the afferent and efferent arterioles
- E  *True.*  Diabetics have an increased susceptibility to bacterial infection leading to both acute and chronic pyelonephritis

# Renal Disease: Questions

85 **Nephrotic syndrome is characterized by:**
   A   Heavy proteinuria
   B   Hypoproteinaemia
   C   Reversed albumin–globulin ratio
   D   Secondary hyperlipidaemia
   E   Oedema

86 **Renal cell carcinoma:**
   A   Is derived from the renal glomerulus
   B   May give rise to polycythaemia
   C   Usually occurs in children under 10 years of age
   D   May invade the renal vein
   E   May present as a pathological fracture

87 **Adult polycystic disease of the kidney:**
   A   Is inherited as an autosomal dominant trait
   B   May be associated with cysts in other organs
   C   Is of no clinical significance
   D   May be associated with subarachnoid haemorrhage
   E   Is frequently associated with mental retardation

88 **Carcinoma of the renal pelvis:**
   A   Is usually squamous in type
   B   May be related to analgesic abuse
   C   Is commonly associated with other tumours in the urinary tract
   D   May be a cause of hydronephrosis
   E   May be associated with renal stones

89 **In renal transplantation:**
   A   An allograft is a transplant from one identical twin to another
   B   Acute rejection of a transplant may be characterized by fibrinoid necrosis of the arterioles of the kidney
   C   Patients receiving immunosuppressive therapy show an increased incidence of malignancy
   D   Patients are susceptible to cytomegalovirus infections
   E   ABO incompatibility would not cause rejection

## Renal Disease: Answers

**85**
- A  *True.*  Usually at least five grammes in 24 hours
- B  *True.*  Due to urinary protein loss
- C  *True.*  Due to depletion of the serum albumin
- D  *True.*  Probably due to synthesis of lipoproteins
- E  *True.*  Generalized oedema is the most obvious clinical manifestation

**86**
- A  *False.*  The tumour originates from the tubular epithelium
- B  *True.*  Due to elaboration of erythropoietin
- C  *False.*  Most commonly seen in late middle-age (40–70 years) with a peak incidence in the sixth decade
- D  *True.*  This is a recognized feature of the tumour which may spread to the inferior vena cava
- E  *True.*  The tumour frequently metastasizes to bone as well as to the lungs, liver and regional nodes

**87**
- A  *True.*  Although about 50 per cent of cases are new mutants
- B  *True.*  Cysts may also be found in the liver, pancreas and lung
- C  *False.*  Many patients develop hypertension and eventual renal failure
- D  *True.*  Berry cerebral aneurysms are found in about 10 per cent of cases
- E  *False.*  There is no relationship between adult polycystic disease and mental retardation

**88**
- A  *False.*  The majority (about 80 per cent) are transitional cell carcinomas
- B  *True.*  There is an increased incidence following analgesic abuse
- C  *True.*  Similar growths may be present in the ureter and bladder
- D  *True.*  Due to urinary outflow obstruction
- E  *True.*  Probably related to chronic irritation

**89**
- A  *False.*  An allograft indicates a donor of the same species but with a different phenotype
- B  *True.*  This is the typical appearance in humoral-type acute rejection
- C  *True.*  Particularly of lymphoma and carcinoma
- D  *True.*  Due to immunosuppressive therapy
- E  *False.*  ABO incompatibility would result in hyperacute rejection

## 90 Carcinoma of the bladder:
A  Is usually squamous in type
B  May be related to schistosomiasis of the bladder
C  Is more common in females than males
D  Has its peak incidence at 35 years of age
E  May be a cause of hydronephrosis

## 91 The following conditions predispose to nephrocalcinosis:
A  Sickle cell disease
B  Multiple myeloma
C  Renal tubular acidosis
D  Lead poisoning
E  Sarcoidosis

## 92 Acute diffuse proliferative glomerulonephritis:
A  Is characterized by increased cellularity of the glomeruli
B  May follow a beta-haemolytic streptococcal throat infection
C  Invariably progresses to a rapidly progressive form
D  May be associated with IgG and complement deposition in the glomeruli
E  Is the most common cause of the nephrotic syndrome in children

## Renal Disease: Answers

**90** A  False.  The majority are transitional cell carcinomas
 B  True.  Schistosomiasis by causing chronic inflammation may predispose to malignancy
 C  False.  More common in males than females in the ratio of about three to one
 D  False.  The disease usually occurs in the 60–70 year-old age group
 E  True.  Due to ureteric obstruction

**91** A  False.  Sickle cell disease predisposes to papillary necrosis, renal infarction and pyelonephritis
 B  True.  The osteolytic lesions may result in hypercalcaemia and deposition of calcium in the kidney
 C  True.  Nephrocalcinosis and stone formation may occur
 D  False.  Lead poisoning may cause tubular defects manifested by glycosuria and aminoaciduria
 E  True.  In this condition there is abnormal sensitivity to vitamin D resulting in hypercalcaemia

**92** A  True.  Largely due to proliferation of mesangial cells. Some neutrophils and eosinophils are also present
 B  True.  Some cases are due to an immune response to a preceding streptococcal infection
 C  False.  Most children with the condition recover. About 50 per cent of adult cases go on to develop chronic disease
 D  True.  IgG and $C_3$ are often found deposited in a granular fashion along the capillary walls and in the mesangium
 E  False.  Most cases are due to the minimal change lesion

# Male and Female Genital Tract Disease

93  Ovarian tumours. Select the *most appropriate* feature listed below which is associated with the tumour:
   A  Granulosa cell tumour
   B  Krukenberg tumour
   C  Brenner tumour
   D  Yolk-sac tumour
   E  Teratoma

   1  Schiller–Duval bodies
   2  Struma ovarii
   3  Donovan bodies
   4  Call–Exner bodies
   5  Signet-ring cells
   6  Touton giant cells
   7  Nests of transitional epithelium in fibrous stroma

94  **Endometrial carcinoma:**
   A  Usually occurs in the 30–40 year-old age group
   B  May be associated with a granulosa cell tumour of the ovary
   C  Usually has an adenosquamous pattern
   D  Typically presents with an abdominal mass
   E  Is more common in multiparous women than nulliparous women

95  **Uterine fibroids:**
   A  Are correctly called fibromyxomas
   B  May undergo rapid growth during pregnancy
   C  Rarely arise before the menopause
   D  Undergo sarcomatous change in about 10 per cent of cases
   E  May undergo calcification

96  **Endometriosis:**
   A  May be a cause of infertility
   B  May cause chocolate cysts in the ovaries
   C  May be a cause of cyclical nose bleeds
   D  Is a recognized cause of dysmenorrhoea
   E  If confined to the ovaries is called adenomyosis

## Male and Female Genital Tract Disease: Answers

**93** A 4    Call–Exner bodies. These are microfollicles of epithelial cells with a central core of eosinophilic material
     B 5    Signet-ring cells. These are mucus-secreting adenocarcinoma cells usually from a primary tumour in the stomach or large intestine
     C 7    Nests of transitional epithelium in fibrous stroma. This is the characteristic histological appearance of this tumour
     D 1    Schiller–Duval bodies. These are glomerular-like perivascular structures
     E 2    Struma ovarii. This is a teratoma consisting almost entirely of thyroid tissue

**94** A False.    This disease usually affects post-menopausal women (average age 55 years)
     B True.    As a result of prolonged oestrogen stimulation
     C False.    About 85 per cent are adenocarcinomas. A very small proportion are adenosquamous and carry a very poor prognosis
     D False.    Irregular uterine bleeding is usually the mode of presentation
     E False.    The condition predominates in unmarried and childless women

**95** A False.    They are leiomyomas. They are composed of smooth muscle often with a slight fibrous tissue component
     B True.    Probably due to stimulation by oestrogen
     C False.    They usually develop during active reproductive life although they may not produce symptoms
     D False.    Sarcomatous change is very rare, probably less than 0·1 per cent of cases
     E True.    When the term 'womb stone' is used

**96** A True.    Due to fibrosis in the Fallopian tubes
     B True.    These are large blood-filled cysts
     C True.    Foci of endometriosis may rarely involve the nasal mucosa
     D True.    Due to intrapelvic bleeding
     E False.    Adenomyosis refers to endometriosis within the myometrium

## Male and Female Genital Tract Disease: Questions

**97 Carcinoma of the uterine cervix:**
- A  Is usually a squamous carcinoma
- B  Is more common in nulliparous women
- C  Metastasizes rapidly to liver and lungs
- D  Almost certainly arises from foci of cervical dysplasia
- E  State II indicates that the tumour is confined to the cervix

**98 In the ovary:**
- A  Serous epithelial tumours have a greater malignant potential than mucinous tumours
- B  Cystic teratomas are usually highly malignant
- C  Ovarian carcinoma is frequently bilateral
- D  Endometrioid tumours may be associated with endometrial carcinoma
- E  Fibromas may be associated with ascites

**99 Hydatidiform mole:**
- A  Only occurs within the uterus
- B  May present with pre-eclampsia
- C  Is associated with raised urinary gonadotrophin levels
- D  Undergoes malignant transformation to a choriocarcinoma in a small percentage of cases
- E  Is usually associated with a normal placenta

**100 Testicular seminoma:**
- A  Usually occurs in elderly men
- B  Arises from the interstitial cells of Leydig
- C  May have a variable lymphocytic infiltrate
- D  Is usually radioresistant
- E  Principally spreads via the lymphatics

**101 Prostatic carcinoma:**
- A  Is usually squamous in type
- B  Frequently metastasizes to bone
- C  May be associated with a raised serum acid phosphatase
- D  Usually responds to treatment with androgens
- E  Usually arises in the lateral lobes

## Male and Female Genital Tract Disease: Answers

**97** A *True.* About 95 per cent squamous; 5 per cent adenocarcinoma
B *False.* More common in married women with children
C *False.* Metastatic spread tends to occur late
D *True.* Almost all cases of carcinoma *in situ* will progress to invasive carcinoma
E *False.* Stage II indicates spread beyond the cervix involving the upper two-thirds of the vagina

**98** A *True.* About 70 per cent of serous tumours are malignant compared with about 30 per cent of mucinous ones
B *False.* The majority of these tumours, also known as dermoid cysts, are benign
C *True.* About 66 per cent of serous cystadenocarcinomas are bilateral
D *True.* About 15–30 per cent are associated with endometrial carcinoma
E *True.* Ascites and pleural effusion (Meigs' syndrome)

**99** A *False.* Rarely, a mole may occur at the site of an ectopic pregnancy
B *True.* This occurs in about 25 per cent of cases
C *True.* The finding of a high HCG level in the urine after the 16th week is suggestive of a mole
D *True.* About 2–3 per cent are followed by the development of a choriocarcinoma
E *False.* There is hydropic swelling of the chorionic villi with associated trophoblastic proliferation

**100** A *False.* About 80 per cent of cases occur in men less than 50 years of age
B *False.* Seminoma arises from the testicular germ cells
C *True.* This is commonly seen and is associated with a better prognosis
D *False.* The tumour is usually radiosensitive
E *True.* Particularly to the para-aortic nodes

**101** A *False.* About 96 per cent are adenocarcinomas usually having a micro-acinar or cribriform appearance
B *True.* Particularly osteosclerotic secondaries in the spine
C *True.* Serum levels greater than 6 i.u. per litre are very suggestive of prostatic carcinoma
D *False.* Androgens probably stimulate tumour growth
E *False.* About 80 per cent arise in the posterior lobe

## 102 Testicular teratoma:
 A  Arises from the interstitial cells
 B  Rarely occurs before the age of 50 years
 C  May produce chorionic gonadotrophin
 D  Carries a better prognosis than the seminoma
 E  Usually spreads to the inguinal nodes

## 103 In the testes:
 A  There is an increased tendency to malignancy in undescended testes
 B  The interstitial cell tumour is usually highly malignant
 C  Viral infection may be a cause of sterility
 D  Seminoma tends to occur at an earlier age than teratoma
 E  Primary lymphoma may occur

## 104 Carcinoma of the penis:
 A  Is usually a transitional cell carcinoma
 B  Has a high incidence among Orthodox Jews
 C  May be related to smegma
 D  Usually arises on the penile shaft
 E  Usually metastasizes to the testes

Male and Female Genital Tract Disease: Answers

**102**  A  False.  It probably arises from the germ cells
     B  False.  About 48 per cent occur in the 20–29 decade
     C  True.   Malignant teratoma trophoblastic (MTT). This worsens the prognosis
     D  False.  The 3-year corrected survival rate for seminoma is 85–90 per cent but only 47 per cent for teratoma
     E  False.  Para-aortic node involvement and blood-spread to the lungs and liver

**103**  A  True.   The risk is 10–40 times greater in the undescended testis
     B  False.  Less than 10 per cent of these Sertoli cell tumours are malignant
     C  True.   Particularly following mumps orchitis
     D  False.  On average the teratoma occurs about 10 years before the seminoma
     E  True.   About 6–7 per cent of testicular tumours are primary lymphomas

**104**  A  False.  The vast majority are squamous carcinomas
     B  False.  The disease is virtually non-existent in this group because circumcision is carried out soon after birth
     C  True.   There is some evidence that smegma may be carcinogenic
     D  False.  The majority occur on the glans or the inner aspect of the prepuce
     E  False.  Spread is usually to the inguinal lymph nodes

# Endocrine Disease

**105 Conn's syndrome:**
A  Is due to oversecretion of antidiuretic hormone
B  May be caused by an adrenal cortical adenoma
C  Is associated with hypokalaemia
D  Is associated with truncal obesity
E  May be a cause of hypertension

**106 Hypoglycaemia is a recognized feature of:**
A  Von Gierke's disease
B  Hepatocellular carcinoma
C  Cushing's syndrome
D  Hypopituitarism
E  Retroperitoneal tumours

**107 The chromophobe adenoma of the pituitary:**
A  Is the most common variety of pituitary tumour
B  May be associated with tumours in other endocrine glands
C  May cause hypogonadism
D  Is associated with Crooke's hyaline degeneration of the chromophobes
E  May cause raised intracranial pressure

**108 The following may occur in primary hyperthyroidism:**
A  Left ventricular hypertrophy
B  Hypercalcaemia
C  Wasting of the muscles
D  Fall in the level of $T_4$ in the blood
E  Exophthalmos

**109 Hashimoto's disease:**
A  Is more common in females than males
B  Is characterized by lymphoid infiltration in the thyroid gland
C  May predispose to the development of thyroid lymphoma
D  Is characterized by massive cervical lymphadenopathy
E  May be associated with the presence of antithyroid antibodies

## Endocrine Disease: Answers

**105** A *False.* The syndrome is due to oversecretion of aldosterone
 B *True.* This is the most common cause. Occasionally it is due to cortical carcinoma
 C *True.* Due to excessive loss of potassium in the urine
 D *False.* Truncal obesity is seen in Cushing's syndrome
 E *True.* Due to sodium retention

**106** A *True.* This glycogen storage disease is due to deficiency of glucose-6-phosphatase
 B *True.* Possibly due to secretion of an insulin-like substance or to excessive utilization of glucose
 C *False.* In Cushing's syndrome, hyperglycaemia and glycosuria may be found
 D *True.* Due to deficiency of growth hormone and ACTH
 E *True.* Particularly retroperitoneal fibrosarcomas

**107** A *True.* It accounts for about two-thirds of pituitary tumours
 B *True.* Adenomas may be found in the pancreas and parathyroids as part of the multiple endocrine adenoma syndrome
 C *True.* Amenorrhoea and sterility in women and impotence and sterility in men
 D *False.* Hyaline degeneration is seen in basophils in association with a basophil adenoma
 E *True.* Due to pressure effects from suprasellar extension of the tumour

**108** A *True.* This may eventually lead to cardiac failure
 B *True.* Due to the catabolic action of thyroid hormone on bone
 C *True.* Thyrotoxic myopathy characterized by muscle wasting and fatty infiltration
 D *False.* The levels of $T_4$ and $T_3$ are usually raised
 E *True.* Due to mucoid oedema of the retro-orbital tissues

**109** A *True.* It is about 12 times more common in females than males
 B *True.* Lymphoid infiltration with follicle formation is seen
 C *True.* Lymphoma develops in the thyroid in a small percentage of cases of Hashimoto's disease
 D *False.* The cervical lymph nodes are not involved
 E *True.* The disease is thought to have an autoimmune aetiology and antibodies to thyroglobulin are usually present

# Endocrine Disease: Questions

**110 In relation to the thyroid:**
A 'Hot' nodules are usually malignant
B Lateral aberrant thyroid is congenitally misplaced thyroid tissue
C Pretibial myxoedema is usually a feature of Hashimoto's disease
D Amyloid may be found in the stroma of thyroid carcinoma
E Long-acting thyroid stimulator may be found in the serum of patients with Grave's disease

**111 Features of Cushing's syndrome include:**
A Osteoporosis
B Relative polycythaemia
C Amenorrhoea
D Hypokalaemia
E Accentuation of the diurnal rhythm of cortisol secretion

**112 The phaeochromocytoma:**
A Is derived from cells of the zona reticularis
B Is usually malignant
C May be found outside the adrenal gland
D May cause elevated vanillylmandelic acid (VMA) levels in the urine
E May be associated with medullary thyroid carcinoma

**113 Addison's disease:**
A May form part of Schmidt's syndrome
B May be an autoimmune disorder
C Is associated with low circulating levels of ACTH
D May cause hypoglycaemia
E Is associated with increased skin pigmentation

**114 Hyperparathyroidism is associated with:**
A Dystrophic calcification
B Metastatic calcification
C Chronic renal failure
D Duodenal ulceration
E Di George syndrome

## Endocrine Disease: Answers

110  A  *False.*  Hot nodules are never malignant. They usually represent functionally autonomous follicular adenomas
    B  *False.*  This represents a metastatic deposit in a lymph node from a primary papillary thyroid carcinoma
    C  *False.*  It is occasionally seen in primary hyperthyroidism (Grave's disease)
    D  *True.*  Amyloid may be found in the stroma of medullary carcinomas
    E  *True.*  This immunoglobulin has a similar effect on the thyroid as thyrotrophin

111  A  *True.*  Due to protein breakdown
    B  *True.*  Due to lowered plasma volume
    C  *True.*  Due to the antagonistic effect of androgens on the endometrium
    D  *True.*  There is sodium retention and increased loss of potassium from the kidney
    E  *False.*  Loss of the diurnal rhythm is a constant finding in the condition

112  A  *False.*  It is derived from the chromaffin cells of the adrenal medulla
    B  *False.*  About 90 per cent are benign
    C  *True.*  For example in the organ of Zuckerkandl
    D  *True.*  VMA is the major breakdown product of catecholamines
    E  *True.*  The phaeochromocytoma may also be associated with neurofibromas and parathyroid adenomas

113  A  *True.*  This is Addison's disease associated with Hashimoto's thyroiditis
    B  *True.*  Many patients have circulating antibodies to adrenal tissue
    C  *False.*  ACTH levels are high due to absence of negative feedback on the pituitary
    D  *True.*  Due to lack of glucocorticoids
    E  *True.*  Possibly due to increased levels of MSH

114  A  *False.*  This refers to calcium deposition in dead tissue when calcium metabolism is normal
    B  *True.*  Elevated serum calcium results in calcification in blood vessels and in the kidneys
    C  *True.*  Renal failure may cause compensatory hyperplasia of the parathyroids
    D  *True.*  Possibly due to calcium deposition in the mucosa of the stomach and duodenum
    E  *False.*  Also known as thymic hypoplasia. In this condition the parathyroids are either hypoplastic or absent

## Endocrine Disease: Questions

**115 In relation to thyroid carcinoma:**
- A  The papillary type usually occurs in the 60–80 year-old age group
- B  There may be an association with radiation to the neck
- C  Psammoma bodies are usually found in follicular carcinoma
- D  Medullary carcinomas may produce calcitonin
- E  Anaplastic carcinoma usually responds to surgical treatment

**116 Aldosterone:**
- A  Is secreted by the zona reticularis of the adrenal cortex
- B  Acts on the distal renal tubule to cause sodium reabsorption
- C  May be secreted by an adenoma of the adrenal cortex
- D  Secretion may be stimulated in liver cirrhosis
- E  May be secreted by pancreatic adenomas

## Endocrine Disease: Answers

**115**
- A  *False.*  Usually seen in females below 40 years of age
- B  *True.*  Radiation is associated with a 50- to 300-fold greater incidence of thyroid carcinoma
- C  *False.*  Psammoma bodies are usually found in papillary carcinomas
- D  *True.*  The parafollicular or C cells may produce calcitonin, ACTH, prostaglandins and serotonin
- E  *False.*  Surgery is usually followed by rapid recurrence and respiratory infection; radiotherapy is the usual method of treatment. The prognosis is poor

**116**
- A  *False.*  Aldosterone is secreted by the zona glomerulosa
- B  *True.*  Sodium is reabsorbed in exchange for potassium or hydrogen ion
- C  *True.*  This is the most common cause of Conn's syndrome
- D  *True.*  Hypoalbuminaemia in cirrhosis causes an increase in extravascular fluid, concurrent hypovolaemia and stimulation of the renin–angiotensin system
- E  *False.*  Although islet cell tumours may secrete other hormones including ACTH, MSH, and HCG

# Bone and Joint Disease

117 **Rheumatoid arthritis:**
   A   May present with hepatosplenomegaly and leucocytosis in children
   B   May be associated with inflammatory changes in the eye
   C   Is characterized by large nodules of collagenous necrosis in the articular cartilage
   D   May be associated with an IgM antibody in the blood
   E   Is not a cause of secondary amyloidosis

118 **Ankylosing spondylitis:**
   A   May be associated with HLA B27 antigen
   B   Characteristically affects adolescent females
   C   May be associated with aortic lesions
   D   Is usually associated with a positive rheumatoid factor
   E   May involve the sacroiliac joints

119 **Paget's disease of bone:**
   A   Is associated with a raised serum alkaline phosphatase
   B   Is characterized histologically by a mosaic cement pattern
   C   Rarely affects the pelvis
   D   May predispose to a chondrosarcoma
   E   May respond to treatment with calcitonin

120 **Osteomalacia:**
   A   May occur in coeliac disease
   B   Is usually associated with normal serum alkaline phosphatase
   C   Is characterized by excessive osteoid formation
   D   May be a complication of antiepileptic treatment
   E   May be associated with areas of osteitis fibrosa cystica in the bones

121 **In fracture repair:**
   A   Poor immobilization may retard healing
   B   Lamellar bone is laid down at the fracture site and is then replaced by woven bone
   C   Union of bone ends by fibrous tissue causes quicker healing than if callus was formed
   D   Changes in pH are important for calcification of osteoid
   E   Cartilage tissue is never formed

## Bone and Joint Disease: Answers

**117**  
A True. Still's disease. The disease often has an acute febrile onset with hepatosplenomegaly, lymphadenopathy and leucocytosis  
B True. Uveitis and keratoconjunctivitis may occur  
C False. The nodules of collagenous necrosis (rheumatoid nodules) are found in the subcutaneous tissues  
D True. This is rheumatoid factor and is found in the serum of about 80 per cent of patients  
E False. RA is one of the most common causes of amyloidosis today  

**118**  
A True. Between 80 and 90 per cent of patients are HLA B27 positive  
B False. Predominantly affects young males between 15 and 35 years of age  
C True. Aortic incompetence occasionally develops in long-standing cases  
D False. This is found in the majority of patients with rheumatoid arthritis  
E True. The sacroiliac, spinal and costovertebral joints are principally affected  

**119**  
A True. Due to increased osteoblastic and osteoclastic activity  
B True. This is pathognomonic of Paget's disease  
C False. The pelvis, skull, spine, femur and tibia are frequently involved  
D False. Paget's may predispose, however, to an osteogenic sarcoma  
E True. Calcitonin acts by reducing osteoclastic activity  

**120**  
A True. Due to failure to absorb vitamin D  
B False. Increased osteoblastic activity causes elevation of alkaline phosphatase  
C True. There is an excess of poorly mineralized osteoid  
D True. Phenobarbitone and phenytoin may impair calcium absorption  
E True. Due to secondary hyperplasia of the parathyroid glands  

**121**  
A True. Rigid immobilization is important for satisfactory fracture healing  
B False. Woven bone is formed first by calcification of osteoid. It is later remodelled to form lamellar bone  
C False. Fibrous union retards proper fracture healing  
D True. Calcium salts are deposited when the pH of the uniting fracture increases (alkaline tide)  
E False. Cartilage tends to form when there is movement at the fracture site

## 122 Osteomyelitis:
A  Rarely involves the metaphysis of the bone
B  May be a cause of amyloid disease
C  May be a cause of squamous carcinoma
D  Is frequently caused by *Staphylococcus pyogenes*
E  May be a cause of Brodie's abscess

## 123 Osteoarthritis:
A  Is a well-recognized cause of amyloidosis
B  Occasionally causes subcutaneous nodules
C  May be associated with Heberden's nodes
D  Mainly affects the synovium
E  Causes an elevated ESR

## 124 Osteogenic sarcoma:
A  Usually occurs at the growing metaphyseal ends of long bones
B  Usually occurs in the first five years of life
C  May result in the radiological feature known as Codman's triangle
D  May be associated with a raised serum alkaline phosphatase
E  Usually metastasizes early to the regional lymph nodes

## 125 Ewing's sarcoma:
A  Rarely occurs before the fifth decade
B  Usually arises from the mid-shaft region of long bones
C  Is characterized by excessive new bone formation by the tumour cells
D  Is characterized by tumour cells containing glycogen
E  May resemble a neuroblastoma

## 126 Osteogenesis imperfecta:
A  May cause fracture formation *in utero*
B  Is inherited as an autosomal dominant condition
C  Is associated with dislocation of the lens
D  Predisposes to osteosarcoma
E  May cause deafness

## Bone and Joint Disease: Answers

**122**  A  False.  The metaphysis is almost always involved
    B  True.  Due to long-standing inflammation
    C  True.  Squamous carcinoma may occur in an inflammatory sinus track between the bone and the skin
    D  True.  This is one of the most common infecting organisms
    E  True.  This is a circumscribed focus of chronic infection

**123**  A  False.  Amyloid is not a complication of this condition which is non-inflammatory
    B  False.  These are a feature of rheumatoid arthritis
    C  True.  These are osteophytes around the terminal interphalangeal joints
    D  False.  The condition is characterized by degeneration of the articular cartilage
    E  False.  The ESR is usually normal

**124**  A  True.  Particularly the lower end of the femur, upper end of the tibia and upper end of the humerus
    B  False.  Most occur between 10 and 30 years of age
    C  True.  There is elevation of the periosteum by the tumour causing a wedge of calcification on X-ray
    D  True.  Due to proliferation of malignant osteoblastic cells
    E  False.  Spread to lymph nodes is not common. Blood-spread, however, occurs to lungs, liver and other bones

**125**  A  False.  The tumour occurs particularly in children and adolescents
    B  True.  Also may occur in the flat bones, such as ribs, vertebrae and pelvis
    C  False.  The tumour cells do not form bone or cartilage
    D  True.  The presence of glycogen in the cells may help in making the diagnosis
    E  True.  A secondary deposit from a neuroblastoma may have a similar histological appearance

**126**  A  True.  Multiple fractures may be present
    B  True.  The bony abnormality may be present at birth or may become apparent during childhood
    C  False.  However, the sclerae are abnormally thin and appear blue
    D  False.  There is no evidence to support this
    E  True.  Due to otosclerosis

## Bone and Joint Disease: Questions

**127 Osteoporosis:**
- A Is characterized by inadequate mineralization of bone
- B Is characterized by a marked fall in serum calcium levels
- C May occur in Cushing's syndrome
- D May predispose to fractures
- E May occur in thyrotoxicosis

**128 The following are recognized causes of hypertrophic osteoarthropathy:**
- A Pleural mesothelioma
- B Osteoarthritis
- C Inflammatory bowel disease
- D Cirrhosis of the liver
- E Asthma

## Bone and Joint Disease: Answers

**127** A  False.  There is an overall loss of bone tissue but what remains shows normal mineralization
  B  False.  Serum calcium is usually normal
  C  True.   Due to excess of adrenocortical hormones
  D  True.   This is an important cause of fractures in elderly people, particularly of the femoral neck
  E  True.   Probably due to exaggerated resorption of bone

**128** A  True.   Mesotheliomas and bronchogenic carcinoma
  B  False.  Although there may be slight swelling at the base of the terminal phalanges of the fingers
  C  True.   Ulcerative colitis and Crohn's disease
  D  True.   Particularly biliary cirrhosis
  E  False.  However, lung sepsis e.g. bronchiectasis and lung abscesses are recognized causes

# Breast and Skin Disease

**129** **In the breast:**
  A  Paget's disease of the nipple is associated only with intraduct carcinoma
  B  Trauma is an important factor predisposing to carcinoma
  C  Lobular carcinoma may be bilateral
  D  Gynaecomastia in males may be the result of liver disease
  E  Apocrine metaplasia is a hallmark of carcinoma

**130** **Carcinoma of the breast:**
  A  Has a higher incidence in multiparous women
  B  Is more common in women with fibrocystic disease of the breast
  C  Usually arises from the ductal epithelium
  D  May be hormone-dependent
  E  Is most commonly found in the lower inner quadrant of the breast

**131** **Carcinoma of the breast:**
  A  Usually presents as bleeding from the nipple
  B  May evoke a desmoplastic reaction
  C  May cause *peau d'orange* of the skin
  D  May respond to treatment with oestrogens
  E  Tends to regress during pregnancy

**132** **Recognized causes of erythema nodosum include:**
  A  Sarcoidosis
  B  Streptococcal infection
  C  Sulphonamides
  D  Inflammatory bowel disease
  E  Amyloidosis

**133** **Squamous cell carcinoma of the skin:**
  A  Is more common in dark-skinned than light-skinned individuals
  B  May histologically resemble a keratoacanthoma
  C  May arise at the site of a chronic skin ulcer
  D  Usually occurs on exposed skin
  E  Usually arises from an intradermal naevus

## Breast and Skin Disease: Answers

**129**  A  *False.*  Intraduct or invasive carcinoma may be present
      B  *False.*  There is no known association between breast carcinoma and trauma
      C  *True.*  Between 10 and 20 per cent are bilateral
      D  *True.*  Liver disease is a recognized cause of hyperestrinism (failure to metabolize oestrogen)
      E  *False.*  This is a benign change seen in large ducts in fibrocystic breast disease

**130**  A  *False.*  More common in nonparous women or those who have their first child after the age of 30 years
      B  *True.*  Carcinoma is about four times more common
      C  *True.*  A small number, however, arise from breast acini (lobular carcinoma)
      D  *True.*  Oestrogen receptors can be identified in cancer cells in about 70 per cent of cases
      E  *False.*  Only about 10 per cent occur here. The majority arise in the upper outer quadrant

**131**  A  *False.*  The majority of cases present as a painless lump
      B  *True.*  This is the formation of a fibrous stroma seen in scirrhous tumours
      C  *True.*  This is characterized by irregular thickening of the skin due to blockage of dermal lymphatics
      D  *False.*  The growth of some breast tumours is enhanced by oestrogens
      E  *False.*  Growth is accelerated during pregnancy

**132**  A  *True.*  This is one of the most common causes in the United Kingdom
      B  *True.*  Including rheumatic fever
      C  *True.*  Other drugs may also cause the condition including penicillin and salicylate
      D  *True.*  Crohn's disease and ulcerative colitis
      E  *False.*  There is no known association between amyloid disease and erythema nodosum

**133**  A  *False.*  Actinic damage to the skin in light-skinned individuals is a predisposing cause
      B  *True.*  Keratoacanthoma is a benign lesion which has a similar histological appearance
      C  *True.*  Chronic inflammation of the skin predisposes to carcinoma, for example in a varicose ulcer
      D  *True.*  The face, neck and hands are most frequently involved
      E  *False.*  It arises from the epidermal squamous epithelium

## Breast and Skin Disease: Questions

**134** Basal cell carcinoma of the skin:
A  Commonly occurs on the face
B  Metastasizes by lymphatics at an early stage
C  Is characterized histologically by keratin pearl formation
D  Is a frequent indicator of an underlying malignancy
E  Usually produces abundant mucin

**135** For the conditions listed select the *most appropriate* skin lesion from those listed below:
A  Rheumatic fever
B  Sarcoidosis
C  Ulcerative colitis
D  Carcinoma of stomach
E  Tuberculosis

1  Lupus pernio
2  Lupus vulgaris
3  Erythema marginatum
4  Acanthosis nigricans
5  Pyoderma gangrenosum
6  Pyogenic granuloma
7  Molluscum contagiosum

**136** Malignant melanoma:
A  Only arises from the skin
B  Is always pigmented
C  Consists of DOPA-positive cells
D  Does not arise in a pre-existing mole
E  Is usually cured by local excision

## Breast and Skin Disease: Answers

**134** A *True.* This is the most common site especially around the eye and the nasolabial folds
B *False.* Metastatic spread of this tumour is extremely rare; it tends to be locally aggressive
C *False.* Keratin pearl formation is a feature of squamous carcinomas
D *False.* There is no relationship between this tumour and an underlying malignancy
E *False.* Mucin production is not a feature of this tumour

**135** A 3 Erythema marginatum. These are discrete circular lesions with raised red margins
B 1 Lupus pernio. These are sarcoid lesions affecting the skin and appear as red plaque-like areas
C 5 Pyoderma gangrenosum. Characterized by ulcerated lesions usually found on the lower limbs
D 4 Acanthosis nigricans. This is darkening and roughening of the skin particularly of the neck, groin and axillae. The condition is associated with an underlying neoplasm
E 2 Lupus vulgaris. This is usually caused by secondary extension of a primary tuberculous lesion or spread via the blood

**136** A *False.* They may arise from the skin, choroid, meninges or conjunctiva
B *False.* Sometimes the tumour shows no pigment—amelanotic melanoma
C *True.* This implies the ability to convert dihydroxyphenylalanine (DOPA) into melanin
D *False.* Most melanomas arise from moles
E *False.* These tumours spread early in the blood and lymphatics

# Nervous System Disease

**137 Medulloblastoma:**
- A  Usually occurs in children
- B  Is usually found in the cerebellum
- C  May result in hydrocephalus
- D  Is not usually radiosensitive
- E  Is derived from the ependyma

**138 Changes in the cerebrospinal fluid in acute bacterial meningitis include:**
- A  Elevated protein
- B  Elevated glucose
- C  Very high lymphocyte count
- D  Luetic Lange's colloidal gold curve
- E  Clear fluid with the formation of a spider-web clot on standing

**139 Multiple sclerosis:**
- A  Has a high incidence in the tropics
- B  Is a cause of optic atrophy
- C  May be associated with a moderate increase in lymphocytes in the CSF
- D  Is characterized by widespread demyelination throughout the grey matter
- E  Usually causes death as a result of raised intracranial pressure

**140 Hydrocephalus is a recognized complication of:**
- A  Arnold–Chiari malformation
- B  Budd–Chiari syndrome
- C  Intrauterine toxoplasmosis
- D  Tuberculous meningitis
- E  Poliomyelitis

**141 Parkinsonism:**
- A  May be due to treatment with phenothiazines
- B  May be caused by manganese poisoning
- C  May follow encephalitis
- D  May be associated with the presence of Lewy bodies in the substantia nigra
- E  Usually responds to treatment with dopamine

## Nervous System Disease: Answers

**137**   A   *True.*   Most cases occur in children less than 14 years of age
       B   *True.*   Usually in the midline
       C   *True.*   Due to extension into the fourth ventricle
       D   *False.*   The tumour is highly radiosensitive
       E   *False.*   Thought to be derived from fetal cells of the external granular layer

**138**   A   *True.*   Due to increased fibrin
       B   *False.*   Sugar is reduced or absent. This is due to utilization by bacteria
       C   *False.*   There is a high polymorph count
       D   *False.*   Lange's colloidal gold curve may be normal or meningitic
       E   *False.*   The fluid is usually turbid or frankly purulent

**139**   A   *False.*   The disease is more common in temperate climates
       B   *True.*   The disease commonly involves the optic nerves
       C   *True.*   These appear to be stimulated T lymphocytes and may represent an immunological response
       D   *False.*   Demyelination occurs in the white matter of the brain and spinal cord
       E   *False.*   Intracranial pressure is normal. Death usually is due to intercurrent infection

**140**   A   *True.*   This is a malformation of the cerebellum with herniation into the cervical spinal canal obstructing CSF flow
       B   *False.*   This is the condition of hepatic vein thrombosis
       C   *True.*   This causes periventricular necrosis in the brain followed by scarring and obstruction to CSF outflow
       D   *True.*   Due to inflammatory adhesions
       E   *False.*   This condition is characterized by destruction of the anterior horn cells of the spinal cord and of brainstem neurones

**141**   A   *True.*   Possibly due to neuronal degeneration in the substantia nigra
       B   *True.*   This causes a progressive Parkinsonian-like syndrome with a coarse tremor
       C   *True.*   Due to damage to the substantia nigra
       D   *True.*   These inclusions are to be found in nearly all cases of primary Parkinson's disease
       E   *False.*   Dopamine will not cross the blood–brain barrier. The precursor L-dopa has to be given

## 142 Subacute combined degeneration of the spinal cord:
A  Usually responds to treatment with folic acid
B  Involves the posterior and lateral columns
C  Principally affects the grey matter
D  Is associated with marked gliosis in the involved areas
E  May be associated with similar degenerative lesions in the brain

## 143 Intracerebral haemorrhage:
A  Is frequently related to hypertension
B  Is usually due to rupture of a berry aneurysm
C  Is frequently due to rupture of the lenticulostriate artery
D  May cause a blood-stained CSF
E  May be associated with an underlying haemorrhagic diathesis

## 144 Spina bifida:
A  May sometimes be diagnosed *in utero* by estimation of alpha-fetoprotein in the amniotic fluid
B  May be associated with the Arnold–Chiari malformation
C  May predispose to meningitis
D  Of the meningocele type is associated with a poorly formed, exposed spinal cord
E  Occulta invariably leads to complete paraplegia

## 145 The astrocytoma:
A  Usually occurs in the cerebellum in adults
B  Usually metastasizes to the cervical lymph nodes
C  May rapidly enlarge due to haemorrhage into the tumour
D  May evoke changes in blood vessels within the tumour
E  Of the type known as glioblastoma multiforme carries the most favourable prognosis

## 146 A cerebral infarct:
A  Typically shows coagulative necrosis
B  Shows accumulation of compound granular corpuscles
C  Involving the basal ganglia may be due to occlusion of the middle cerebral artery
D  Is a well-recognized complication of myocardial infarction
E  Is almost always pale in type

## Nervous System Disease: Answers

**142**
- A  False.  Administration of vitamin $B_{12}$ is required. The anaemia, however, may respond to folate
- B  True.  Usually the posterior columns first
- C  False.  The condition is one of demyelination and affects the white matter
- D  False.  There is little reactive gliosis
- E  True.  Foci may appear in the cerebral white matter causing confusion and dementia

**143**
- A  True.  This is the most important predisposing factor
- B  False.  Rupture of a berry aneurysm usually results in subarachnoid haemorrhage
- C  True.  This leads to haemorrhage in the internal capsule area
- D  True.  Due to blood leaking into the ventricular system
- E  True.  Such as leukaemia or thrombocytopenic purpura

**144**
- A  True.  Raised levels of alpha-fetoprotein in amniotic fluid may indicate an open neural tube defect
- B  True.  In this condition there is herniation of the cerebellum into the spinal canal
- C  True.  If the meninges are exposed and not protected in the spinal canal
- D  False.  In a meningocele the cord is usually normal. The defect is herniation of the meninges
- E  False.  There is usually only occasional minor neurological abnormality

**145**
- A  False.  In adults it is usually found in the cerebral hemisphere. Cerebellar astrocytomas occur in children
- B  False.  Extra-cranial metastasis of gliomas is rare
- C  True.  This may cause acute deterioration in the patient's condition causing acute hemiplegia
- D  True.  Endothelial hyperplasia, thrombosis and lymphocytic cuffing are associated with the higher grades of this tumour
- E  False.  This is the most anaplastic variant of astrocytoma and carries the worst prognosis

**146**
- A  False.  Liquefactive or colliquative necrosis is typically seen
- B  True.  These cells, also known as Gitter cells, are microglial cells containing abundant lipid
- C  True.  This is the most common site of cerebral infarction
- D  True.  Either due to embolism from a mural thrombus or as a result of hypotension following cardiogenic shock
- E  False.  Many cerebral infarcts, especially of embolic origin, are haemorrhagic

**147 Chronic subdural haematoma:**
- A Is more common at the extremes of life
- B May follow a trivial head injury
- C May be associated with fluctuation in clinical signs
- D Usually undergoes a progressive reduction in size
- E Is usually caused by rupture of a 'berry' aneurysm on the circle of Willis

**148 Meningiomas:**
- A Usually occur in children under five years of age
- B Are more common in women than men
- C May invade the skull
- D Histologically may show the presence of psammoma bodies
- E Arise from the Purkinje cells in the cerebellum

## Nervous System Disease: Answers

**147**  A  *True.*  Infants and old people are particularly susceptible
    B  *True.*  In many instances, no history of trauma is available, presumably because a trivial injury had been overlooked
    C  *True.*  This makes diagnosis difficult
    D  *False.*  The haematoma tends to enlarge, possibly as a result of osmosis or continued slow bleeding
    E  *False.*  It is probably due to rupture of bridging veins crossing the subdural space

**148**  A  *False.*  They occur in adult life (usually 45–55 years of age)
    B  *True.*  In a ratio of 2:1
    C  *True.*  This may result in the formation of a hyperostosis
    D  *True.*  These are spherical laminated calcified particles
    E  *False.*  The tumour arises from the arachnoid cells

# Haematology

149 **Chronic myeloid leukaemia:**
   A  Is rare in children
   B  Is characterized by massive lymph node enlargement
   C  Is associated with high neutrophil alkaline phosphatase
   D  Is associated with the Philadelphia chromosome
   E  Usually only causes very slight elevation of the white cell count

150 **Multiple myeloma:**
   A  May cause a leucoerythroblastic anaemia
   B  Is associated with the excretion of IgG in the urine which may be precipitated by heating
   C  May result in amyloidosis
   D  May result in marked rouleaux formation on a peripheral blood film
   E  Causes renal failure in a high proportion of cases

151 **Erythrocytosis:**
   A  May be caused by uterine fibroids
   B  May present with myocardial infarction
   C  Usually causes a fall in serum uric acid
   D  May progress to leukaemia
   E  Causes marked elevation of serum alkaline phosphatase

152 **Leucoerythroblastic anaemia:**
   A  Is characterized by the presence of immature red and white cells in the peripheral blood
   B  May occur in myelofibrosis
   C  May be associated with metastatic carcinoma in bone
   D  May be associated with benzene poisoning
   E  May occur in chronic heart failure

153 **In sickle cell anaemia:**
   A  Most adult patients develop massive splenomegaly
   B  Crisis may be precipitated by acidosis
   C  There is increased susceptibility to pneumococcal infections
   D  Extramedullary haemopoiesis does not occur
   E  Leg ulcers are frequently seen in adults

## Haematology: Answers

**149**
- A  *True.*  It usually occurs in the 40–50 year-old age group
- B  *False.*  Hepatosplenomegaly is present but lymph node enlargement is not usually significant
- C  *False.*  Leukaemic granulocytes have low levels of alkaline phosphatase
- D  *True.*  About 95 per cent of cases are associated with part of the long arm of chromosome 22 translocated to chromosome 9
- E  *False.*  White cell count is usually very high 100–400 × 10$^9$ per litre

**150**
- A  *True.*  This is characterized by the appearance of immature red and white cells in the blood
- B  *False.*  Bence–Jones protein is composed of monoclonal light chains
- C  *True.*  This develops in about 10 per cent of cases
- D  *True.*  Due to raised plasma protein
- E  *True.*  Due to blockage of the tubules by protein casts

**151**
- A  *True.*  Due to inappropriate erythropoietin production
- B  *True.*  Due to increased risk of thrombosis
- C  *False.*  This is usually raised due to increased red cell turnover
- D  *True.*  Erythrocytosis may progress to myelosclerosis or myeloblastic leukaemia
- E  *False.*  However, neutrophil alkaline phosphatase is increased

**152**
- A  *True.*  This is the characteristic picture in this condition
- B  *True.*  Associated with progressive fibrosis of the marrow
- C  *True.*  Associated with extensive replacement of bone marrow by tumour
- D  *True.*  Due to the toxic effects of benzene on the bone marrow
- E  *False.*  There is no association between the two conditions

**153**
- A  *False.*  The spleen becomes shrunken due to repeated infarction (autosplenectomy)
- B  *True.*  Sickling is enhanced by an acid pH
- C  *True.*  Possibly related to an impairment of the alternative complement pathway normally activated by bacterial polysaccharide
- D  *False.*  Haemopoiesis may appear in the spleen and liver
- E  *True.*  Due to vascular stagnation in the subcutaneous tissues

## Haematology: Questions

**154 Acute lymphoblastic leukaemia:**
- A Usually develops in childhood
- B May be associated with chromosomal abnormalities
- C Does not affect the central nervous system
- D May cause splenomegaly
- E Carries a better prognosis in males than females

**155 Hereditary spherocytosis:**
- A May be associated with the formation of gallstones
- B Is inherited as a sex-linked recessive characteristic
- C May cause splenomegaly
- D Is due to glucose-6-phosphate dehydrogenase deficiency
- E May be complicated by acute marrow aplasia

**156 Splenomegaly is a feature of:**
- A Gaucher's disease
- B Tay–Sachs disease
- C Felty's syndrome
- D Brucellosis
- E Typhoid fever

**157 Concerning lymphomas:**
- A Most non-Hodgkin's lymphomas arise from B cell lymphocytes
- B There may be an association with the Epstein–Barr virus
- C Mycosis fungoides is a lymphomatous condition involving the skin
- D Hodgkin's disease is more common in females than males
- E Are usually associated with a 'leukaemic' type blood picture

**158 In Hodgkin's disease:**
- A Warthin–Finkeldey cells are usually found in involved lymph nodes
- B Stage II disease indicates involvement of lymph node regions on both sides of the diaphragm
- C The mixed cellularity type carries the best prognosis
- D Lacunar cells may be found
- E There may be impairment of T lymphocyte function

## Haematology: Answers

**154**
- A True. This is the commonest form of leukaemia in children
- B True. There is an increased incidence in Down's syndrome
- C False. Leukaemic cells may be found in the meninges
- D True. There may be enlargement of the liver, spleen and lymph nodes
- E False. Prognosis is worse in males compared with females because of recurrence of leukaemia in the testes

**155**
- A True. Due to increased breakdown of red cells
- B False. The condition is inherited in an autosomal dominant fashion
- C True. The spleen is hyperplastic
- D False. The condition is due to a defect in the red cell membrane
- E True. The hyperplastic marrow is susceptible to aplastic failure particularly following infections

**156**
- A True. Due to accumulation of glucocerebrosides in lymphoreticular cells
- B False. Accumulation of ganglioside occurs only in nerve cells
- C True. A form of rheumatoid arthritis characterized by lymphadenopathy and splenomegaly
- D True. Focal granulomata are found in the spleen
- E True. Localization of *Salmonella typhi* occurs in the lymphoreticular tissues

**157**
- A True. About 68 per cent arise from B cell lymphocytes
- B True. This virus is causally related to Burkitt's lymphoma
- C True. This is a primary lymphoma of the skin
- D False. Males are affected about twice as frequently as females
- E False. There is no significant spill-over of lymphoma cells into the peripheral blood until a late stage in the disease

**158**
- A False. These are giant cells found in measles infection
- B False. Stage II indicates involvement of two or more lymph node regions on the same side of the diaphragm
- C False. Lymphocyte predominant carries the most favourable prognosis (70 per cent 10 years survival)
- D True. These are variants of Reed–Sternberg cells and are usually found in nodular sclerosing Hodgkin's disease
- E True. Patients with Hodgkin's disease have an increased susceptibility to fungal infections and to tuberculosis and they also show impaired rejection of skin grafts

## 159 Classical haemophilia:
A Causes prolongation of the bleeding time
B Is inherited as an autosomal recessive condition
C Causes prolongation of the kaolin–cephalin clotting time (partial thromboplastin time)
D May result in joint deformity in adults
E Is due to deficiency of factor IX

## 160 Infectious mononucleosis (glandular fever):
A May be a cause of splenic rupture
B May cause hepatitis
C Is thought to be caused by a herpes virus
D Is associated with heterophile antibodies in the serum
E May be associated with atypical lymphocytes in the blood

**159**  A  False.  Bleeding time is normal since platelet activity is normal
    B  False.  It is inherited as an X-linked recessive condition
    C  True.   This tests the intrinsic clotting system
    D  True.   Due to repeated bleeding into the joints
    E  False.  There is deficiency of factor VIII. Christmas disease is deficiency of factor IX

**160**  A  True.   The spleen is enlarged and its capsule is weakened due to infiltration with lymphocytes
    B  True.   Infiltration with lymphocytes and mononuclear cells is seen in the liver with foci of liver cell necrosis
    C  True.   The Epstein–Barr virus
    D  True.   These will agglutinate sheep red cells (Paul–Bunnell test)
    E  True.   These are T lymphocytes

# Miscellaneous

161 **Carcinoid tumour of the ileum:**
   A   Virtually never metastasizes
   B   May be a cause of intestinal obstruction
   C   Is derived from APUD cells
   D   May produce 5-hydroxyindoleacetic acid
   E   Has a better prognosis than carcinoid of the colon

162 **In chronic bronchitis:**
   A   E. Coli can usually be cultured from the sputum
   B   Bronchial mucous glands undergo atrophy
   C   Left ventricular hypertrophy usually occurs
   D   Sulphur dioxide in the atmosphere may be an important aetiological factor
   E   There may be associated emphysema of the lungs

163 **The following predispose to acute pyelonephritis:**
   A   Vesicoureteric reflux
   B   Benign nodular hyperplasia of the prostate
   C   Simple cysts of the renal cortex
   D   Pregnancy
   E   Catheterization

164 **Ulceration of the intestinal mucosa typically occurs in:**
   A   Tuberculous enteritis
   B   Regional ileitis
   C   Giardiasis
   D   Coeliac disease
   E   Amoebic dysentery

165 **Sudden unexpected death is a recognized feature of:**
   A   Hypertrophic obstructive cardiomyopathy
   B   Calcific aortic stenosis
   C   Sarcoidosis of the heart
   D   Viral myocarditis
   E   Floppy mitral valve syndrome

## Miscellaneous: Answers

**161**    A    False.    Carcinoid of the appendix virtually never metastasizes, but the same is not true in the ileum
        B    True.    Due to fibrosis of the bowel wall and peritoneal adhesions
        C    True.    This refers to amine precursor uptake decarboxylation, a function of the cells
        D    False.    It produces 5-hydroxytryptamine which is excreted in the urine as 5HIAA
        E    False.    Colonic carcinoids are usually benign and hormonally inactive

**162**    A    False.    The organisms most commonly found are *Haemophilus influenzae* and pneumococci
        B    False.    There is hyperplasia of mucous glands
        C    False.    Right ventricular hypertrophy leading to cor pulmonale is a feature
        D    True.    Sulphur dioxide is a potent irritant of the bronchial mucosa
        E    True.    Most patients show evidence of both conditions hence the use of the term chronic obstructive airways disease

**163**    A    True.    Reflux allows ascent of organisms from the bladder to the kidney
        B    True.    Prostatic enlargement may cause urinary tract obstruction and urinary retention
        C    False.    These have no functional significance and do not predispose to infection
        D    True.    Due to pressure on the ureters from the enlarged uterus
        E    True.    By introducing organisms from the urethra into the bladder

**164**    A    True.    Circumferential ulcers of the terminal ileum occur
        B    True.    In Crohn's disease there is mucosal ulceration and transmural inflammation
        C    False.    Giardiasis may however cause villous atrophy and malabsorption
        D    False.    This causes villous atrophy
        E    True.    Undermined flask-shaped ulcers in the pelvic colon and caecum

**165**    A    True.    Possibly due to abnormality of the conduction system although this has not been definitely proven
        B    True.    Due to inadequate coronary artery perfusion
        C    True.    Usually due to involvement of the conducting system
        D    True.    This predisposes to the development of arrhythmias, e.g. ventricular fibrillation
        E    True.    Possibly due to upward ballooning of the valve

## Miscellaneous: Questions

**166 Minimal change glomerulonephritis:**
- A Is rare in adults
- B Usually presents as hypertension
- C Shows no glomerular abnormality on light microscopy
- D Shows lumpy deposition of immune complexes on the glomerular basement membrane on immunofluorescence
- E Has a poor prognosis

**167 In benign essential hypertension:**
- A Most patients die of renal failure
- B The majority of patients have high circulating levels of renin
- C Hyaline arteriolosclerosis is seen in the kidneys
- D Adrenal hyperplasia occurs in long-standing cases
- E Progression to an accelerated phase may occur

**168 Polyarteritis nodosa:**
- A May be a cause of coronary thrombosis
- B Is associated with fibrinoid necrosis of the artery walls
- C May be caused by sulphonamides
- D May involve the renal glomerulus
- E Is usually associated with raised levels of anti-mitochondrial antibodies

**169 A list of tumours and anatomical sites is given. Select the *most appropriate* site for each of the five tumours listed:**
- A Craniopharyngioma
- B Brenner tumour
- C Diktyoma
- D Cystosarcoma phylloides
- E Chemodectoma

1. Ovary
2. Testis
3. Kidney
4. Eye
5. Breast
6. Carotid body
7. Pituitary

## Miscellaneous: Answers

**166**
- A True. Most cases occur in children between 1 and 6 years of age
- B False. The condition usually presents as the nephrotic syndrome
- C True. Usually no abnormality can be detected on light microscopy
- D False. Immunofluorescence shows no immune deposits
- E False. With treatment the long-term prognosis is good

**167**
- A False. Most patients die from cardiac failure. Only about 5 per cent develop renal failure
- B False. High plasma renin is found in only about 15 per cent of patients
- C True. Hyaline arteriolosclerosis is the hallmark of essential hypertension although it may occur in other conditions
- D False. The adrenals show no abnormality
- E True. A few patients progress to accelerated or malignant hypertension characterized by fibrinoid necrosis of arterioles

**168**
- A True. Due to arteritis affecting the coronary vessels
- B True. Fibrinoid necrosis associated with inflammation in the vessel wall
- C True. A number of drugs have been implicated including sulphonamides, iodides and aspirin
- D True. Patchy necrosis of the glomerular tuft may occur
- E False. There is no definite evidence of an autoimmune origin and the condition probably represents a hypersensitivity reaction in the vessel wall

**169**
- A 7 Pituitary. The tumour arises from vestigial remnants of Rathke's pouch
- B 1 Ovary. This tumour is characterized by nests of epithelial cells in a fibrous stroma
- C 4 Eye. This tumour arises from the epithelium of the ciliary body
- D 5 Breast. Also known as a giant fibroadenoma of the breast. Most are benign but a small percentage undergo sarcomatous change
- E 6 Carotid body. This tumour arises from non-chromaffin paraganglia

Miscellaneous: Questions 85

**170 In coarctation of the aorta:**
A  The segment of narrowing is usually proximal to the origin of the innominate artery
B  The blood pressure in the legs is decreased
C  Infection may occur at the site of the coarctation
D  There is usually marked cyanosis in the 'adult' type
E  Aneurysmal dilation of the aorta may occur

**171 Match the organism with the *most appropriate* condition in the list below:**
A  Lymphogranuloma venereum
B  Hydatid disease
C  Q fever
D  Choroidoretinitis
E  Food poisoning

1  *Coxiella burnettii*
2  *Cryptococcus neoformans*
3  *Ascaris lumbricoides*
4  *Salmonella typhimurium*
5  Chlamydia
6  *Echinococcus granulosus*
7  *Toxoplasma gondii*

**172 Recognized features of pernicious anaemia include:**
A  Antibodies to gastric parietal cells
B  An association with Hashimoto's disease
C  Autosomal dominant inheritance
D  Increased risk of developing gastric carcinoma
E  Leucocytosis

**173 Anaphylaxis:**
A  Is an example of cell-mediated hypersensitivity
B  Is usually mediated by IgG
C  Is associated with degranulation of mast cells
D  May be characterized by acute bronchospasm
E  Occurs in the Arthus reaction

## Miscellaneous: Answers

**170** A  False.  The coarctation is between the left subclavian artery and the site of the ductus arteriosus
  B  True.  An increased blood pressure is found in the head, neck and arms
  C  True.  Infection at this site is similar to that seen in infective endocarditis
  D  False.  Cyanosis does not occur because there is no shunting of blood
  E  True.  An aneurysm may form above or just below the coarcted segment

**171** A  5  Chlamydia. LGV is a venereal disease characterized by ulcerated genital lesions and lymphadenopathy
  B  6  *Echinococcus granulosus*. Hydatid disease is characterized by cysts in the liver. The dog is the definite host
  C  1  *Coxiella burnettii*. Q fever usually causes an influenza-like illness often with patchy consolidation of the lungs
  D  7  *Toxoplasma gondii*. Toxoplasmosis may affect the eyes in both the congenital and adult forms of the disease
  E  4  *Salmonella typhimurium*. The organism is a common cause of food poisoning often due to eating contaminated poultry or their eggs

**172** A  True.  Found in 80–90 per cent of patients. Also antibodies to intrinsic factor may be present
  B  True.  Both conditions are thought to have an autoimmune aetiology
  C  False.  There may be a family history of PA but no definite mode of inheritance is known
  D  True.  Associated with atrophic gastritis and intestinal metaplasia
  E  False.  Neutropenia is usual. The neutrophils show nuclear hypersegmentation

**173** A  False.  Anaphylaxis is a type I immediate hypersensitivity reaction mediated by immunoglobulin
  B  False.  It is due to IgE
  C  True.  Causing the release of histamine, serotonin, slow-reacting substance and heparin
  D  True.  Due to smooth muscle contraction in bronchial walls
  E  False.  This is due to antigen–antibody complex formation

## Miscellaneous: Questions

**174** The following may be associated with diabetes:
- A  Increased incidence of atheroma
- B  Renal papillary necrosis
- C  Increased incidence of infection
- D  Nephrotic syndrome
- E  Underweight newborn infants

**175** In chronic cholecystitis:
- A  The gallbladder is usually palpable
- B  Gallstones are usually present
- C  Sinuses may be present in the gallbladder wall
- D  There is an association with infertility
- E  There is an increased incidence of carcinoma of the gallbladder

**176** The following are more common in females than males
- A  Carcinoma of the rectum
- B  Turner's syndrome
- C  Systemic lupus erythematosus
- D  Paget's disease of bone
- E  Grave's disease

**177** Phaeochromocytoma:
- A  Usually arises from the adrenal cortex
- B  Is usually benign
- C  May be associated with thyroid cancer
- D  May be a cause of left ventricular hypertrophy
- E  Usually produces serotonin

**178** Lymph node hyperplasia may occur in:
- A  Infectious mononucleosis
- B  Chronic pruritic skin disease
- C  Asbestosis
- D  Hypothermia
- E  Patients taking phenytoin

## Miscellaneous: Answers

**174**    A    *True.*    The aorta and medium-sized arteries show severe atheromatous change
       B    *True.*    Possibly due to microangiopathy
       C    *True.*    Particularly skin infections and pyelonephritis
       D    *True.*    Due to diffuse glomerulosclerosis
       E    *False.*    Infants of diabetic mothers tend to be overweight

**175**    A    *False.*    The gallbladder is usually contracted
       B    *True.*    Stones are usually found in about 90 per cent of cases
       C    *True.*    These are protrusions of epithelium into the muscle and serosa
       D    *False.*    No such association is known
       E    *True.*    Probably related to chronic irritation from stones and inflammation

**176**    A    *False.*    More common in males than females in a ratio of 2:1
       B    *True.*    This is usually associated with a single X chromosome (45 XO)
       C    *True.*    This autoimmune disease is about 10 times more common in females than males
       D    *False.*    This condition has a slight male preponderance
       E    *True.*    The condition is about 5 times more common in females than males

**177**    A    *False.*    The adrenal medulla is the most common site. A few arise outside the adrenal gland
       B    *True.*    Only about 5–10 per cent are malignant
       C    *True.*    Medullary carcinoma of the thyroid
       D    *True.*    As a result of an elevated blood pressure
       E    *False.*    Catecholamines, particularly noradrenaline

**178**    A    *True.*    The lymph nodes may be enlarged and painful. The spleen is also enlarged
       B    *True.*    This is known as dermatopathic lymphadenopathy
       C    *False.*    The lymph nodes are not involved in this condition
       D    *False.*    Lymph node enlargement has not been described in hypothermia
       E    *True.*    Phenytoin may cause lymphadenopathy, arthropathy and hepatosplenomegaly

## 179 Left ventricular hypertrophy:
A  Is best determined by direct weighing of the separated left ventricle
B  May occur with aortic coarctation
C  May occur with an adrenal cortical adenoma
D  Does not occur in the cardiomyopathies
E  Is associated with increase in the total number of myocardial fibres

## 180 Congenital pyloric stenosis:
A  Presents as projectile vomiting about 3 days after birth
B  Is more common in males than females
C  Is due to hypertrophy of the pyloric muscle
D  May be cured by Ramstedt's operation
E  May be associated with degenerative changes in the ganglion cells of Auerbach's plexus

## 181 Scleroderma (systemic sclerosis):
A  May be associated with Raynaud's phenomenon
B  May be a cause of dysphagia
C  May cause decalcification of bones
D  Is not associated with a rise in antinuclear antibodies
E  May cause renal failure

## 182 The following conditions show an X-linked recessive mode of inheritance:
A  Congenital pyloric stenosis
B  Huntington's Chorea
C  Christmas disease
D  Marfan's syndrome
E  Polycythaemia vera

## Miscellaneous: Answers

**179** A  True.   This is the most accurate method. Measurement of the thickness of the left ventricular wall, although routinely carried out, is somewhat inaccurate
  B  True.   Due to narrowing of the aorta with resistance to left ventricular outflow
  C  True.   If it secretes cortisol or aldosterone resulting in a raised blood pressure
  D  False.  Hypertrophy is an important feature of cardiomyopathy and is particularly marked in the hypertrophic obstructive type (HOCM)
  E  False.  Hyperplasia indicates increase in the number of fibres. Hypertrophy implies increase in size of the individual fibres

**180** A  False.  Symptoms usually occur about 3 weeks after birth
  B  True.   About 85 per cent of infants affected are boys
  C  True.   There is hypertrophy of the circular muscle forming the pyloric sphincter
  D  True.   This operation involves splitting the muscle coat down to the mucosa
  E  True.   The number of ganglion cells is reduced and degenerative changes have been noted

**181** A  True.   The combination of Raynaud's and scleroderma is termed acrosclerosis
  B  True.   Due to fibrosis of the oesophageal wall
  C  True.   Due to immobilization by the stiffened skin
  D  False.  Titres of antinuclear antibodies are high as in systemic lupus erythematosus
  E  True.   Involvement of the renal vasculature occurs and may progress to renal failure

**182** A  False.  Inheritance in this condition appears to be multifactorial
  B  False.  This condition, characterized by atrophic changes in the brain, has an autosomal dominant mode of inheritance
  C  True.   A bleeding disorder due to deficiency of factor IX
  D  False.  Inheritance in this condition is autosomal dominant
  E  False.  No mode of inheritance is known although the condition is more common in members of the same family

## 183 Diarrhoea is a recognized feature of:
A Verner–Morrison syndrome
B Myxoedema
C Carcinoid syndrome
D Diabetes
E Medullary carcinoma of thyroid

## 184 Thromboangitis obliterans:
A Mainly affects arterioles
B Is more common in men than women
C May also affect veins and nerves
D May be a cause of gangrene
E May be aggravated by smoking

## 185 Phenylketonuria:
A Is inherited as a sex-linked recessive condition
B May be diagnosed by estimating the salt content of sweat
C Is due to deficiency of the enzyme phenylalanine hydroxylase
D May cause mental retardation
E Rarely causes symptoms before 5 years of age

## 186 There is a recognized association between:
A Silicosis and bronchial carcinoma
B Silicosis and tuberculosis
C Oat-cell carcinoma of the lung and Cushing's syndrome
D Smoking and alveolar cell carcinoma
E Haematite and bronchial carcinoma

## 187 Acquired immunodeficiency syndrome (AIDS):
A Occurs exclusively among male homosexuals
B Appears to have a long incubation period
C May be associated with the development of Kaposi's sarcoma
D Is thought to be caused by *Listeria monocytogenes*
E Appears to be spread by droplet infection

## Miscellaneous: Answers

**183**  
A True. Due to an islet-cell tumour producing vasoactive intestinal peptide (VIP)  
B False. These patients often have constipation  
C True. Due to secretion of 5-hydroxytryptamine  
D True. Due to autonomic neuropathy  
E True. Thought to be due to secretion of prostaglandins by the tumour  

**184**  
A False. The condition affects medium-sized arteries  
B True. The vast majority of cases occur in men, usually between the ages of 20 and 40 years  
C True. The inflammation may involve the entire neurovascular bundle  
D True. The condition affects limb vessels and thrombosis may result in gangrene, especially in the legs  
E True. Possibly due to the vasoconstrictive effect of tobacco smoking  

**185**  
A False. The mode of inheritance is autosomal recessive  
B False. Diagnosis is by detection of phenylpyruvic acid in the urine or by estimation of phenylalanine in the blood  
C True. Lack of this enzyme causes accumulation of phenylalanine in the blood  
D True. Cerebral damage is thought to be due to high circulating levels of phenylalanine or its metabolites  
E False. Symptoms of instability, vomiting and fits develop in the first few weeks of life  

**186**  
A False. There is no evidence that silicosis predisposes to lung cancer  
B True. Silicosis predisposes to pulmonary tuberculosis  
C True. Due to ectopic ACTH production by the tumour  
D False. Smoking predisposes to the development of bronchial tumours (usually squamous and oat-cell types)  
E True. There is an increased incidence of lung cancer in haematite miners  

**187**  
A False. The condition is also recognized as occurring in Haitians and haemophiliacs  
B True. Possibly several years  
C True. This is a malignant vascular tumour usually occurring in the skin of the limbs  
D False. The cause of the condition is unknown but is thought to possibly be a virus  
E False. Infection is acquired through sexual contact and from infected blood products

## 188 In Crohn's disease:
A There may be submucosal fibrosis in the terminal ileum
B Malabsorption may be a complication
C Intestinal obstruction is a recognized complication
D There may be an association with ankylosing spondylitis
E Fistulae rarely occur

## 189 Amniotic fluid embolism:
A Cannot occur without rupture of the membranes
B Is usually associated with a uterine tear
C Is a recognized cause of sudden death during labour
D May be detected by histological examination of the lungs
E Is a recognized complication of laparoscopic sterilization

## 190 Diverticular disease:
A Most commonly affects the rectum
B May be associated with Marfan's disease
C May result in a vesicocolic fistula
D May be a cause of melaena
E Is thought to be due to atrophy of the circular muscle of the bowel wall

## 191 Stein–Leventhal syndrome:
A Is characterized by multiple luteal cysts in the ovary
B May cause virilization
C Is associated with a cortical adrenal adenoma
D Is a form of ovarian endometriosis
E May cause infertility

## Miscellaneous: Answers

**188** A  True.   Fibrosis is particularly marked in the submucosa
B  True.   Widespread inflammation and mucosal ulceration may result in malabsorption of fat, vitamin $B_{12}$, protein and electrolytes
C  True.   Due to stricture formation caused by thickening of the bowel wall
D  True.   Crohn's disease may be associated with a number of conditions including AS, iridocyclitis, cirrhosis and polyarthritis
E  False.  Fistulae are a well-recognized complication, particularly following surgery

**189** A  True.   The membranes must be broken to allow communication between the fluid and maternal venous channels
B  True.   Particularly small incomplete tears in the lower uterine segment
C  True.   Shock with profound hypotension is a recognized feature
D  True.   The presence of fetal squames, vernix, meconium and lanugo hairs may be seen in the pulmonary vessels
E  False.  Air embolism may, however, occur during this procedure

**190** A  False.  The rectum is never involved. The sigmoid colon is most commonly affected
B  True.   There may be a connective tissue defect in the bowel wall
C  True.   A pericolic abscess may erode into the bladder wall. Gas and faeces may enter the bladder
D  True.   Due to ulceration of the mucosa within inflamed diverticula
E  False.  The circular muscle is much thicker and has a corrugated appearance

**191** A  False.  Multiple follicular cysts are found
B  True.   Due to increased secretion of androgens from the ovaries and possibly the adrenals
C  False.  The adrenals are usually histologically normal
D  False.  The condition is not related to endometriosis which is characterized by ectopic foci of endometrial glands and stroma in the ovary
E  True.   This may respond to treatment with clomiphene

## Miscellaneous: Questions

**192 In ischaemic colitis:**
A The sigmoid colon is most commonly involved
B Strictures may occur
C Mucosal ulceration is unusual
D There may be segmental involvement of the bowel
E Fistula formation is common

**193 Select the most appropriate histological stain for the material from the list below:**
A Neutral fat
B Melanin
C Calcium
D Fibrin
E Plasma cells

1 Congo red
2 Unna–Pappenheim
3 Masson–Fontana
4 Lendrum's MSB
5 Periodic acid Schiff
6 von Kossa
7 Oil red O

**194 Deficiency of:**
A Thiamine causes beri-beri
B Nicotinic acid causes pellagra
C Calciferol causes hypercalcaemia
D Pyridoxine causes a megaloblastic anaemia
E Ascorbic acid causes scurvy

**195 Thymus-dependent lymphocytes:**
A In the spleen are principally found in the red pulp
B In lymph nodes are mainly found in the germinal centres
C Are important in cell-mediated immunity
D Are plasma cell precursors
E Produce immunoglobulin

**196 Giant cell (temporal) arteritis:**
A Only involves the cranial vessels
B Is thought to be caused by tight-fitting headwear
C May be associated with polymyalgia rheumatica
D May be a cause of cerebral infarction
E Usually occurs in young adult male smokers

## Miscellaneous: Answers

**192**  A  *False.*  The splenic flexure is most frequently affected
 B  *True.*  Characterized by granulation tissue formation and subsequent fibrosis in the submucosa
 C  *False.*  Mucosal ulceration is a constant feature
 D  *True.*  Short segments of the bowel may be affected with normal bowel at each end of the diseased area
 E  *False.*  Fistulae do not occur in this condition

**193**  A  7  Oil red O. This stains fat red in frozen sections
 B  3  Masson–Fontana. This stains melanin pigment dark-brown to black
 C  6  von Kossa. This stains calcium deposits black
 D  4  Lendrum's MSB. This stains fibrin red although 'old' fibrin may appear bluish
 E  2  Unna–Pappenheim. This stains the DNA and RNA in these cells

**194**  A  *True.*  Characterized by neurological lesions and cardiac arrhythmias
 B  *True.*  Characterized by diarrhoea, dermatitis and dementia
 C  *False.*  Calciferol deficiency will cause osteomalacia and rickets
 D  *False.*  Deficiency may cause a hypochromic, microcytic anaemia
 E  *True.*  Characterized by a bleeding tendency and poor wound healing

**195**  A  *False.*  The white pulp contains the lymphocyte population
 B  *False.*  They are found in the paracortical areas
 C  *True.*  This is an important function of the cells
 D  *False.*  It is thought that B lymphocytes are plasma cell precursors
 E  *False.*  Virtually all circulating antibodies are produced by plasma cells

**196**  A  *False.*  The lesions may also involve the aorta and its branches
 B  *False.*  This was suggested in the past but is now thought to be untrue
 C  *True.*  This condition is characterized by diffuse symmetrical muscle pain and stiffness
 D  *True.*  Due to cerebral artery thrombosis
 E  *False.*  It tends to occur in the older age group (usually over 60 years) and is slightly more common in females

## Miscellaneous: Questions

**197 Duchenne-type muscular dystrophy:**
- A  Is inherited as an autosomal recessive condition
- B  May eventually involve the respiratory muscles
- C  Is associated with raised serum creatine kinase levels
- D  Mainly involves the proximal muscle groups
- E  Is characterized histologically by an inflammatory cell reaction in the affected muscles

**198 Gout:**
- A  Is usually associated with raised blood uric acid levels
- B  Is characterized by precipitation of calcium pyrophosphate in the joints
- C  May occur secondary to cytotoxic therapy for cancer
- D  Frequently involves the metatarsophalangeal joint of the great toe
- E  May cause impairment of renal function

**199 Haemolytic uraemic syndrome:**
- A  Usually occurs in infants and young children
- B  Is associated with thrombocytopenia
- C  Is characterized by microthrombi in the renal arterioles and glomerular capillaries
- D  Is associated with deposition of immunoglobulins and complement in the glomeruli
- E  May be associated with schistocytes in the peripheral blood

**200 Features of secondary syphilis include:**
- A  Snail-track ulcers
- B  Positive Wassermann reaction
- C  Maculopapular rash
- D  Aortitis
- E  Gumma formation

## Miscellaneous: Answers

**197** A  False.  The disease is inherited as a sex-linked recessive characteristic
    B  True.  This is the usual reason for death
    C  True.  This is useful for diagnosis and for detecting carriers
    D  True.  The proximal limb muscles are particularly involved
    E  False.  No inflammatory reaction is present. There is loss of muscle fibres and fatty infiltration

**198** A  True.  The serum uric acid level is usually greater than 0·4 mmol/litre
    B  False.  Calcium pyrophosphate is deposited in the joints in pseudogout. The plasma urate level is normal in pseudogout
    C  True.  Due to increased nuclear breakdown
    D  True.  Although other joints such as the knee, elbow and finger joints may be involved
    E  True.  Due to deposition of urate crystals in the kidney

**199** A  True.  Most cases occur between 6 and 18 months of age
    B  True.  Anaemia, reticulocytosis and thrombocytopenia occur
    C  True.  These changes are seen in the early stage of the disease
    D  False.  These have not been demonstrated in glomeruli
    E  True.  These are fragmented red cells damaged in the haemolytic process

**200** A  True.  These occur on the buccal and pharyngeal mucosa
    B  True.  A positive WR is invariably found
    C  True.  Particularly on the palms of the hands and soles of the feet
    D  False.  This is a feature of the tertiary stage and may cause aortic incompetence and aneurysm formation
    E  False.  These are foci of granulation tissue formation with central necrosis and occur in the tertiary stage